10 Powerful Ideas for Improving Patient Care: Book 3

Your board, staff, or clients may also benefit from this book's insight. For more information on quantity discounts, contact the Health Administration Press Marketing Manager at (312) 424-9470.

Reprinted September 2014

Library of Congress Cataloging-in-Publication Data
Bisognano, Maureen A.
    10 powerful ideas for improving patient care. Book 3 / Maureen Bisognano and Robert Lloyd.
        p.   cm.
    Includes bibliographical references.
    ISBN-13: 978-1-56793-266-9
    ISBN-10: 1-56793-266-5
        1. Medical care—Quality control.   I. Lloyd, Robert C.   II. Title.   III. Title: Ten powerful ideas for improving patient care.

    RA399.A1B58 2006
    362.1—dc22

                                                                                        2006049614

The paper used in this publication meets the minimum requirements of American National Standard for Information Sciences—Permanence of Paper for Printed Library Materials, ANSI Z39.48-1984.™

Project manager: Jane Calayag; Acquisitions editor: Audrey Kaufman; Cover designer: Trisha Lartz

Health Administration Press
A division of the Foundation of the
    American College of Healthcare Executives
1 North Franklin Street, Suite 1700
Chicago, IL 60606-3424
(312) 424-2800

Institute for Healthcare Improvement
20 University Road, 7th Floor
Cambridge, MA 02138
(617) 301-4800

Introduction

This is the third book in the series entitled *10 Powerful Ideas for Improving Patient Care,* designed to widely share innovations in patient care and operational processes in both inpatient and outpatient settings.

In June 2006, Don Berwick, president and chief executive officer of the Institute for Healthcare Improvement (IHI), announced that during the past 18 months more than 3,100 hospitals across the United States prevented approximately 122,000 avoidable patient deaths (IHI 2006). The hospitals accomplished this feat by participating in IHI's 100,000 Lives Campaign—an initiative aimed at creating a new standard of healthcare by introducing six proven patient-care interventions and asking U.S. hospitals to immediately implement these practices in their institutions.

The success of the Campaign demonstrates that significant improvements in care can be achieved quickly and broadly, a fact that goes against research indicating that best practices typically remain on the shelf for 17 years before they are adopted widely enough to directly benefit patients (Landro 2005). The Campaign's broad coalition of care sites, partners, and donors also shows that the healthcare industry can unite to effect profound change. As Cleve Killingsworth (2006), president and chief executive officer of Blue Cross Blue Shield of Massachusetts, wrote in an op-ed piece, "the wind of reform [is] at our backs."

FINDING GOOD IDEAS AND IMPLEMENTING THEM NOW

For this book, authors Maureen Bisognano and Robert Lloyd assembled a new set of ideas that will help leaders and frontline staff improve the care at their organizations. The suggestions detailed in this book are reliable, innovative, ready for testing or implementation, and have been vetted and used successfully in local areas; references for each idea are given so that your team can follow up for further information.

Research at IHI demonstrates a strong link between introducing innovation and improving both quality and staff morale. Improvement often happens at a frustratingly slow pace; however, a devotion to testing new changes regularly and repeatedly will quicken the pace of improvement. Often, staff morale dramatically increases and turnover decreases as facilities adopt innovative improvements and spread them across the organization.

SPREADING CHANGES THROUGHOUT THE ORGANIZATION

IHI's Leadership Model and A Framework for Spread are critical approaches to accelerating improvement and spreading changes.

The Leadership Model, created by Tom Nolan (2000) and later expanded by IHI (Reinertsen, Pugh, and Bisognano 2003), identifies the core set of activities that leaders must engage in to produce a shared mission, vision, and values (along with will, ideas, and organizational processes) that drive improvement.

A Framework for Spread, also developed by IHI (Schall et al. 2006), has helped IHI plan and execute the diffusion of new ideas and new performance levels, both within an organization and between similar systems. In our experience, complete and reliable spread across all organizational units happens only when leaders drive the process, often guided by a model such as A Framework for Spread.

We urge you to consider the lessons from the 100,000 Lives Campaign as you think about improvement throughout your organization. One of these lessons is that there is a tremendous amount of will within the healthcare community to change the system for the better. The ideas presented in this book can help you harness that will and create the kind of unprecedented improvements that hospitals and other care sites are achieving all over the world.

WHY THESE IDEAS?

To determine which ideas would be included in this book, we asked ourselves the following questions:

- Would we want to use this idea in our own organizations?

- Does this idea have appeal for leaders at multiple levels in an organization, from the chief executive officer to frontline managers?
- Does this idea have appeal across multiple clinical and professional disciplines?
- Does this idea have the potential to truly transform practices or to go beyond merely incremental improvement?
- Does this idea hold the potential to make processes and care better for patients and families?
- Is this idea being used?

Ideas that passed the test—that is, for which all answers to these questions were "yes"—became prime candidates for inclusion.

HOW TO USE THIS BOOK

Each chapter provides a description of the idea, an example of the idea in practice, and, in most cases, the results that have been achieved when the idea was applied.

Leaders may use this book in a variety of ways. Some may read it straight through, getting an overview of all ten ideas and thinking broadly about how the ideas may fit into their organizational strategies. Others may want to zero-in on the ideas that hold particular relevance

for their organizations. We encourage readers to choose whatever approach suits them. Our hope is that these ideas lead to action: Pick one, two, or all ten, and then try them out. Ask yourself, as we are fond of saying at IHI, "What can I do by next Tuesday?"

WHERE TO LEARN MORE

- To learn more about IHI's 100,000 Lives Campaign, including "How-to Guides" for implementing all six interventions, visit www.ihi .org/IHI/Programs/Campaign/.
- For more information on leadership for improvement and spreading changes, see the following white papers:

  - "Seven Leadership Leverage Points for Organization-Level Improvement in Health Care" at www.ihi.org/IHI/Results/White Papers/SevenLeadershipLeverag ePointsWhitePaper.htm.
  - "A Framework for Spread: From Local Improvements to System-Wide Change" at www.ihi.org/IHI/Results/White Papers/AFrameworkforSpread WhitePaper.htm.

The first two books in this series offer more ideas:

- Reinertsen, J. L., and W. Schellekens. 2004. *10 Powerful Ideas for Improving Patient Care.* Chicago: Health Administration Press and the Institute for Healthcare Improvement.

- Bisognano, M., and P. Plsek. 2006. *10 More Powerful Ideas for Improving Patient Care.* Chicago: Health Administration Press and the Institute for Healthcare Improvement.

REFERENCES

Institute for Healthcare Improvement. 2006. "IHI Announces That Hospitals Participating in 100,000 Lives Campaign Have Saved an Estimated 122,300 Lives." [Online information; retrieved 9/8/06.] www.ihi.org/NR/rdonlyres/1C51BADE-0F7B-4932-A8C3-0FEFB654D747/0/UPDATED100kLivesCampaignJune14milestonepressrelease.pdf.

Killingsworth, C. 2006. Opinion-Editorial. *Boston Globe* (June 21): 95.

Landro, L. 2005. "Informed Patient: Healthcare Quality Programs Under Fire." *The Wall Street Journal* (July 6): D1.

Nolan, T. 2000. "A Primer on Leading Improvement in Healthcare." Presented at the Fifth European Forum on Quality Improvement in Health Care, Amsterdam, March 24.

Reinertsen, J. L., M. D. Pugh, and M. Bisognano. 2005. "Seven Leadership Leverage Points for Organization-Level Improvement in Health Care." Cambridge, MA: Institute for Healthcare Improvement.

Schall, M. W., M. R. Massoud, G. A. Nielsen, K. Nolan, and C. Sevin. 2006. "A Framework for Spread: From Local Improvements to System-Wide Change." Cambridge, MA: Institute for Healthcare Improvement.

Use Early-Detection and Monitoring Systems

C ardiac arrests are usually preceded by observable signs of deterioration, often six to eight hours before the arrest occurs. Early recognition of these signs and prompt treatment can reduce death rates in hospitalized patients. One of the six patient-care interventions recommended by the Institute for Healthcare Improvement (IHI) through its groundbreaking 100,000 Lives Campaign is for hospitals to establish rapid response teams. A rapid response team—also known as a medical emergency team or MET—is a group of clinicians who bring critical care expertise to the patient bedside, or wherever needed. Implementing such a team is the subject of Idea 5 in *10 More Powerful Ideas for Improving Patient Care* (Bisognano and Plsek 2006).

The idea of using early-detection and monitoring systems is based on research indicating that patients often exhibit signs and symptoms of increasing instability (e.g., changes in breathing, heart rate, or mental status) several hours before a critical event (e.g., heart attack). Early detection allows patients to be rescued early in their decline before a potential crisis occurs. ▶

NEEDED: MORE RELIABLE MONITORING SYSTEMS

Current methodologies for monitoring and detecting signs of patient deterioration have not changed much since they were designed more than a century ago by Florence Nightingale. Although taking a patient's blood pressure, pulse, respiration, and temperature remains the backbone of monitoring systems and protocols, new methods and systems are needed. According to DeVita (2005), "Hospitals in the future must develop methodologies to find more reliably [those] patients who are in crisis, and then respond to them swiftly and effectively to prevent unnecessary deaths."

Why are more reliable methods for identifying a potential patient crisis necessary? Take a look at the current conditions faced by nurses and physicians working in medical-surgical units:

- From 1980 to 2001, the average length of stay in hospitals declined from 7.3 days to 5.0 days (Hall and DeFrances 2003).
- Patient-turnover rates have increased to as high as 40 percent to 50 percent of the midnight census (Norrish and Rundall 2001).

- Nurses spend 13 percent to 28 percent of their shifts documenting patient care (Korst et al. 2003; Pabst, Scherubel, and Minnick 1996; Smeltzer et al. 1996; Upenieks 1998).
- In 2004, the total time all healthcare workers (not just nurses) spent providing direct patient care and assessment on a medical-surgical unit was an average of 1.7 hours during a 12-hour period (*Quality Letter for Healthcare Leaders* 2004).

These statistics paint a clear picture: Patient turnover is increasing, but the time spent administering direct patient care (including monitoring patients for signs of distress) is decreasing. In addition, patient acuity has increased, requiring shorter lengths of stay, and more minor procedures are being performed in ambulatory settings. These realities underscore the need to redesign processes for observing, monitoring, and triggering responses for patients in distress.

PATIENT AND FAMILY INVOLVEMENT

Although there are specific recommended criteria for calling a team, most rapid response teams in hospitals are designed to be activated by anyone, even by patients or their family members. This is only logical given that, often, patients and their family are the first to identify early signs of distress and deterioration.

Tamra Merryman, R.N., FACHE, a quality improvement vice president at the University of Pittsburgh Medical Center (UPMC) Shadyside Hospital, is a champion of patient and family involvement in care. UPMC, in collaboration with Sorrel King—founder of the Josie King Foundation and mother of 18-month-old Josie who died as a result of a medical error—has developed a new monitoring and response tool called Condition H (the H stands for help).

Condition H is a rapid response team that can be triggered by patients and their family members as well as by staff. Upon admission, all patients and family members are trained on how to use Condition H. As of the end of 2005, Condition H was used five times, and each of these calls was later evaluated to be appropriate. The development of Condition H not only represents an improvement of an existing monitoring and response system, it also demonstrates the importance and power of patient and family involvement when redesigning care systems.

OTHER INNOVATIVE APPROACHES

At Seton Northwest Hospital, a central-Texas facility in the Ascension Health network, providing appropriate training to the nursing staff is key to the hospital's ability to identify signs of patient distress. This approach is based on an important nursing philosophy: Every patient deserves an experienced nurse, and every new nurse deserves an experienced nurse. The nursing staff perform regular rounds on their units. During these rounds, an advanced practice nurse accompanied by a less-experienced nurse checks on every patient to assess changes in status and to detect early signs of a deteriorating condition. The advanced practice nurse trains the less-experienced nurse on how to identify distress signs during these rounds. Together, both nurses develop more sophisticated early warning criteria to make their rapid-response process even more reliable. In addition to receiving training on detection, newer nurses also learn advanced communication skills, which are essential to the effectiveness of a detection and rapid-response system.

More inventive methods come from Carol Haraden, Ph.D., vice

president at IHI; John Whittington, M.D., medical director and patient safety officer at OSF Saint Francis; and their colleagues at the Safer Patients Initiative based in the United Kingdom. The group has developed sophisticated early warning systems that reliably identify patients in trouble and that trigger the appropriate, often life-saving response. Whittington (2005) points out two essential elements of a reliable early warning system:

1. It should be simple and practical, using routine physiological measurements and observations that identify the patient's risk.
2. It should facilitate the timely attendance to the patient by members of the care team who possess the appropriate skills, knowledge, and experience.

Single-Parameter System

The most basic type of an early warning system is the so-called "single-parameter system," which relies on periodic observation of selected vital-sign values (e.g., heart rate, blood pressure, urinary output). In this system, when one or more extreme values are noted (e.g., extreme elevation in blood pressure), a predefined action is taken and the rapid response team is called. Figure 1.1 shows a simple example of a single-parameter early warning system; note the first criterion in this example: Staff member is worried about the patient. Mere concern for a patient should—and, in this system, will—trigger the response. Instinct plays a part in the decision to trigger a rapid response team, as discussed in Idea 5 of *10 More Powerful Ideas for Improving Patient Care* (Bisognano and Plsek 2006).

Another tool developed at the Luton and Dunstable Hospital NHS Trust in the United Kingdom is a color-coded chart that makes the decision to call for help easy for the observing caregiver. When any one of the vital signs being recorded (e.g., temperature, pulse, blood pressure, respiration) falls into the red zone, the nurse (or caregiver) is prompted to call the rapid response team. This tool has increased the ease, speed, and reliability of identifying at-risk patients and has ensured timely responses from physicians or outreach nurses.

Multiple-Parameter System

This detection system is based on a regular review of selected vital signs. It directs a caregiver to take action

Figure 1.1. Single Parameter Early Warning System

Adult Rapid Response Team Criteria

- Staff member is worried about the patient
- Acute change in heart rate <40 or >130 bpm
- Acute change in systolic blood pressure <90 mmHg
- Acute change in respiratory rate <8 or >28 per minute or threatened airway
- Acute change in saturation <90% despite oxygen administration
- Acute change in conscious state
- Acute change in urine output to <50 ml in 4 hours

Source: Reprinted with permission from Institute for Healthcare Improvement, Cambridge, Massachusetts.

when any two of the patient's vital signs become cause for concern; Figure 1.2 shows an example of a multiple-parameter system. Note the first of the two instructions at the bottom of Figure 1.2: "If a patient fulfills *two or more* of the above criteria *OR* you are worried about his/her condition, page the resident from the admitting team and the rapid response team."

This system is not meant to undercut the capability of, or to replace the autonomy of, the individual caregiver, who relies on his experience and unique skill set. Rather, it is designed to augment the caregiver's experience and skill set, giving him support in detecting patients who are at risk.

Aggregate-Weighted Scoring System

The final type of warning system is the aggregate-weighted scoring system. Just as the single- and multiple-parameter systems do, this system relies on the observation of preselected basic vital signs. The difference here is that the entire assessment is scored, and if that score exceeds a previously agreed-on threshold, the appropriate action is triggered. Figure 1.3 shows an example of an aggregate-weighted scoring system from the Burton Hospitals NHS Trust in the United Kingdom. Shown in the figure is a modified, simple design of the system, where the preselected vital signs are listed in the left-most

Figure 1.2. Multiple-Parameter Early Warning System

- Systolic blood pressure   <101   >200
- Respiratory rate   <9   >20
- Heart rate   <51   >110
- Saturation (room air)   <90%
- Urine output   <1ml/kg/2 hours
- Conscious level   Not fully alert

- If a patient fulfills *two or more* of the above criteria *OR* you are worried about his/her condition, page the resident from the admitting team and the rapid response team.
- These two parties <u>must</u> review the patient *within thirty minutes.*

Source: Reprinted with permission from Barking, Havering, and Redbridge Hospitals NHS Trust, Romford, Essex, England.

column and the scoring ranges are listed across the top. Each of the vital signs is assigned a value range, and this range correlates to a score. For example, heart rate in the range of 101–110 is assigned a score of 1; blood pressure of less than 30 percent below the normal patient value is assigned a score of 2. At the bottom of the figure, the threshold trigger level is identified. When a specific vital sign reaches the trigger level or exceeds the value range, the caregiver must call the rapid response team.

An advantage of this system is that it can be automated; in fact, some hospitals already have such an automated system. With an automated system, the values for the vital signs are entered into the electronic medical record system. When the values hit or exceed the trigger threshold, the system is prompted to call for help. Again, this automation is meant to serve as an additional level of reliability; it is not meant to replace the decision-making ability of the caregiver or care team.

CONCLUSION

The implementation of rapid response teams is gaining momentum in hospitals worldwide. For these teams to be most effective, proper

Figure 1.3. Modified Aggregate-Weighted Scoring System Tool

MEWS Score Table: Queens Hospital, Burton Hospitals, NHS Trust

Score	3	2	1	0	1	2	3
RR		<8		9–14	15–20	21–29	>30
HR		<40	40–50	51–100	101–110	111–129	>130
BP	<45%	<30%	<15%	Normal for pt.	>15%	>30%	>45%
CNS				Alert	Responds to voice	Responds to pain	Unresponsive
Temp		<35.0%		35–38.4		>38.4	
Urine		<.05 ml/kg/hr	<1 ml/kg/hr		>3 ml/kg/hr		

Trigger level: Score 4 for surgical patients with an adjustment for medical patients.
Key: RR: respiratory rate; HR: heart rate; BP: blood pressure; CNS: mental status; Temp: temperature; Urine: urinary output

Source: Reprinted with permission from Burton Hospitals NHS Trust, Burton-on-Trent, Staffordshire, England.

systems are needed for identifying which patients are most at risk and when they reach their critical points. Only a few innovative approaches for such a monitoring and detection system are mentioned in this chapter. We hope that these examples will generate new ideas.

WHERE TO LEARN MORE

- Establishing a rapid response team is one of the six interventions recommended by IHI's 100,000 Lives Campaign. For more information, including the "How-to Guide," visit www.ihi.org/ihi/Programs/Campaign/Campaign.htm?TabId = 2.
- To learn more about the Safer Patients Initiative in the United Kingdom, visit www.ihi.org/IHI/Programs/SaferPatients Initiative/.
- Learn more about the Josie King Foundation at www.josieking.org.

REFERENCES

Bisognano, M., and P. Plsek. 2006. *10 More Powerful Ideas for Improving Patient Care.* Chicago: Health Administration Press and the Institute for Healthcare Improvement.

DeVita, M. 2005. "Medical Emergency Teams: Deciphering Clues to Crises in Hospitals." *Critical Care* 9 (4): 325-26.

Hall, M. J., and C. J. DeFrances. 2003. 2001 *National Hospital Discharge Survey. Advance Data from Vital and Health Statistics*, No. 332. Hyattsville, MD: National Center for Health Statistics. [Online information; retrieved 6/15/06.] www.cdc.gov/nchs/data/ad/ad332.pdf.

Korst, L. M., A. C. Eusebio-Angeja, T. Chamorro, C. E. Aydin, and K. D. Gregory. 2003. "Nursing Documentation Time During Implementation of an Electronic Medical Record." *Journal of Nursing Administration* 33 (1): 24-30.

Norrish, B. R., and T. G. Rundall. 2001. "Hospital Restructuring and the Work of Registered Nurses." *Milbank Quarterly* 79 (1): 55-79, IV.

Pabst, M. K., J. C. Scherubel, and A. F. Minnick. 1996. "The Impact of Computerized Documentation on Nurses' Use of Time." *Computers in Nursing* 14 (1): 25-30.

Quality Letter for Healthcare Leaders. 2004. "Keeping Patients Safe: Institute of Medicine Looks at Transforming Nurses' Work Environment." *Quality Letter for Healthcare Leaders* 16 (1): 9-11.

Smeltzer, C. H., P. A. Hines, H. Beebe, and B. Keller. 1996. "Streamlining Documentation: An Opportunity to Reduce Costs and Increase Nurse Clinicians' Time with Patients." *Journal of Nursing Care Quality* 10 (4): 66-77.

Upenieks, V. V. 1998. "Work Sampling. Assessing Nursing Efficiency." *Nursing Management* 29 (4): 27-29.

Whittington, J. 2005. Personal communication, November 3.

Develop a Culture Capable of Achieving Organizational Objectives

A considerable amount of discussion about culture can be heard these days. People are talking about "a culture of quality," "a culture of safety," "the organization's leadership culture," and "service excellence culture," to name a few. There are formal cultures, and then there are informal cultures, the most powerful type of culture. "Culture" is a term that is tossed around a great deal, begging the important but little-asked question: "What is culture?"

Classic textbook definitions of culture include a group's established norms, or the behavioral expectations for members of a group, or even a group's social ▶

mores. In most healthcare organizations, however, when staff reflect about the culture they usually think about a very simple definition: a culture developed in the lab to test for the presence of bacteria. *Taber's Cyclopedic Medical Dictionary* (1983, 354), for example, defines culture as "The propagation of microorganisms or of living tissue cells in a special medium that is conducive to growth." Following this definition, without a medium for growth, a culture cannot develop or flourish. This logic is just as true of a bacteria culture placed in a Petri dish as it is of the more amorphous concept of organizational culture.

A MEDIUM FOR GROWTH

Apply this culture-growth analogy to your own organization. What mediums for growth of organizational culture are in place? Do these mediums produce cultures that may be considered "good" or "bad"? The simple answer is that cultures are neither good nor bad. For example, the culture of a monastic order has a very different set of objectives from the culture of a group of thieves. A culture that is effective (or "good") for thieves (e.g., a culture that fosters lying and cheating) would

consider the culture of monks (e.g., a culture that embraces meditation) to be diametrically opposed to the thieves' own objectives and therefore is unacceptable (or "bad").

The effectiveness of a culture is best determined when this is considered: Is the culture capable of achieving the objectives of the organization? Note that many people think they do not have the ability to effect changes within their culture. However, the simple truth is that members of a culture can make an impact on their culture, but first members have to understand the factors that form and then drive the culture. In short, you need to gain knowledge of how to create mediums for growth of an effective culture.

FOUR COMPONENTS OF CULTURE

A culture that is effective and allows the organization to achieve its stated objectives does not develop by chance. It also does not develop merely because your organization won a quality award two years ago or has a nicely worded vision statement. An effective culture is the product of a deliberate focus on four basic components, shown in Figure 2.1.

Figure 2.1. Organizational Components of an Effective Culture

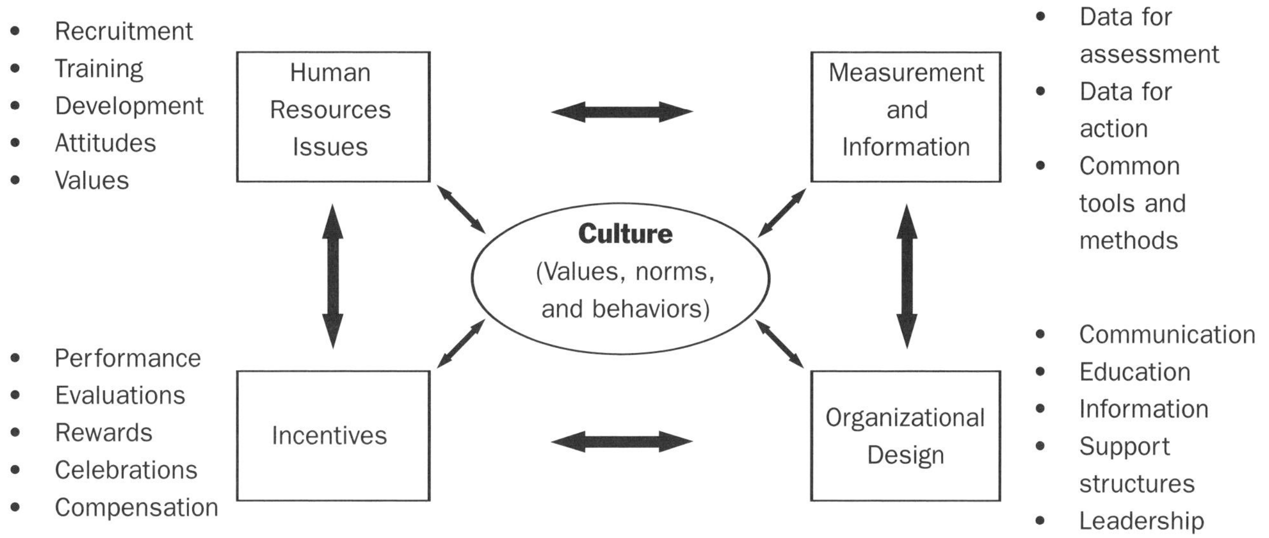

- Recruitment
- Training
- Development
- Attitudes
- Values

Human Resources Issues

Measurement and Information

- Data for assessment
- Data for action
- Common tools and methods

Culture
(Values, norms, and behaviors)

- Performance
- Evaluations
- Rewards
- Celebrations
- Compensation

Incentives

Organizational Design

- Communication
- Education
- Information
- Support structures
- Leadership

Source: Reprinted with permission from R. C. Lloyd and Associates.

Human Resources

The first component relates to human resources issues—who we hire, how we train them, and what we do to retain them. If employees are our most valuable resource (which almost every organization says at one point or another), then a considerable amount of our effort ought to be directed at this component. Many healthcare organizations screen job applicants, to allow them to see the applicants' alignment with the organizational culture. Disney and Southwest Airlines are two well-known companies that use initial screenings to determine alignment between potential employees and the organizational mission, values, and philosophy. Southwest refers to its process as "Targeted Selection." Central to Southwest's selection process are the candidate's humor and the extent to which the candidate seems capable of becoming part of an extended family of people who work hard and have fun at the same time (Freiberg and Freiberg 1996, 67). With use of a screening tool, if an applicant does not meet certain criteria of the organization, she is told this up front, preventing waste of the person's and the company's time.

Another key human resources consideration relates to retention of good staff. Again, most organizations state, "Our employees are our most valuable resource!" Yet, when you look at the retention rates of these organizations and the basis on which they reward employees and build employee loyalty, you frequently wonder why any employee stays with these organizations. W. Edwards Deming (2000, 53) put it this way: "The greatest waste in America is failure to use the abilities of people." This statement is true in many healthcare organizations.

Why do some people love going to work each day, and why do others hate to get out of bed and face another day on the job? One reason relates to the fair and competitive wages some employees receive, but that is only part of the equation. The other part, which is a major factor in the healthcare industry, has nothing to do with salary or perquisites. It is related to how employees are treated, how they feel about their coworkers, their respect for their managers, and the opportunities they have for self-expression and meaningful work. This valuable part links to organizational leadership and how these leaders create incentives for their most valuable resource.

Incentives

What motivates healthcare workers? Why do they enter this profession? The typical response to these questions is, "I wanted to help people." Rarely do you hear that the primary motivators are financial bonuses and stock options. Money is certainly a key motivator of any job, but for healthcare workers (especially those in not-for-profit organizations) other factors (e.g., achievement, recognition, responsibility, work itself) also seem to be perceived as major incentives (Herzberg 2003). Organizations that do not give serious consideration to factors that motivate their employees will never be able to develop and sustain an effective culture.

Organizational Design

An organization's structural design is the result of a direct and purposive set of decisions made by the leadership of the organization. Central in these decisions are the ways in which the following functions are designed and deployed:

- Education of staff and management
- Communication, including both the actual content of the information and the ways in which it is disseminated

- Information flow, including the amount that is shared with employees as well as the types of information shared
- Support structures for providing patient care, including the admitting and scheduling processes and the physical layout of the office space
- Leadership structures, including the number of formal leaders, their ranges of responsibility, and their abilities to manage complex systems

Healthcare is not known for its innovative approaches to management and change. Organizational and professional hierarchies are quite strong in this industry and play dominant roles in healthcare delivery and decision making. The hierarchies within the ranks of physicians, nurses, and administrators did not happen by accident; leaders of the organization created them. They are frequently perpetuated by the rigid structure of the organization with its multilayered reporting relationships. Although we allow such structures to continue by following them, most healthcare professionals complain regularly about the lack of flexibility and innovation afforded by these organizational designs.

Measurement and Information

Organizational measurement can be classified into two basic categories: (1) measurement of the voice of the customer (i.e., finding out what the wants, needs, and expectations of the customers really are) and (2) measurement of the voice of the process (i.e., collecting data to understand the variation that exists in the processes and outcomes that customers experience). Within each of these categories, management and staff must decide how they will assess performance and how they will use the collected data to make improvements. Using the right tools and techniques to understand the variation that exists in processes is vital. Good measurement begins with having an overall philosophy and approach toward measurement and monitoring. Doing what has always been done and measuring what has always been measured will not contribute to the organization's long-term survival.

These four components—human resources, incentives, organizational design, and measurement and information—are the key ingredients for creating an effective culture. People often view organizations as the collection of physical structures and tangible assets, but the truth is that people and culture are the essence of organizations. This is most likely why Deming (1993) listed psychology (or human behavior) as one of the four key components of his concept of "profound knowledge."

Individuals with hopes, wishes, aspirations, and desires are the basis of organizational culture. It is the people who build the cultures. How organizational leaders choose to manage and build this culture will determine the organization's fate. Unfortunately, many leaders do not think about the cultures they are creating, allowing cultures to emerge, grow, and change on their own. They often view building and maintaining a culture as the "soft side of healthcare" and not as easy to influence as the financial aspects of the business ("the hard side"). It is incumbent on leaders, however, to study the components of creating effective cultures.

EXAMPLE: ASCENSION HEALTH

Many examples exist of how healthcare organizations have taken a deliberate and concerted approach to understanding the mediums for culture growth that they have put in place. James Reinertsen, M.D., (2005), a Senior Fellow at IHI, captured the essence of organizational culture this way: "I think the most important bit to know is that there isn't one culture in any organization—there are scores of microcultures, clustered around supervisors, managers, [and] microsystems. When you work on improving culture, you don't work on it in the same way across the entire organization, but you custom-craft your approach to each of the microcultures."

Ascension Health in St. Louis, Missouri, embodies Reinertsen's comments. The organization has developed a precise and comprehensive process—the Safety Climate Survey—to gather data on the cultures that exist across its 68 hospitals and 890 clinical units. David Pryor, M.D., Ascension's senior vice president of clinical excellence and the senior sponsor for cultural transformation at Ascension, clearly understands the impact of culture on the organization. He lives by the perspective that "culture eats strategy for lunch." Pryor's assumption suggests the interplay that exists between culture and strategy. In addition, Pryor argues that an organization can make an impact on the culture on three levels: the hospital level, the unit level, and the individual level. To achieve this, however, leaders need to understand the current status of the culture and then develop changes that will modify the mediums for growth (Pryor 2005).

Ascension's Safety Climate Survey is a step in this direction, providing leaders an opportunity to think about unit-level cultures. Developed by Bryan Sexton and colleagues at the Johns Hopkins University in Baltimore, Maryland, the survey was first administered at Ascension in the summer and fall of 2004 to all staff (including nonemployed physicians) involved in clinical activities. Thus far, more than 30,000 surveys have been completed, providing the organization with baseline data and the potential framework for understanding the many cultures that exist throughout the Ascension system. The survey was repeated in early 2006 to determine the degree of cultural change that has occurred. Comparative reports are now being developed by Pryor and his staff.

Results from the completed surveys indicate a considerable variation across the hospitals with respect to a culture of teamwork, with 50 percent to 80 percent of respondents reporting a positive teamwork culture. When the results were broken out over 890 units, the variation ranges from 17 percent to 100 percent of respondents reporting a positive teamwork climate. These results point leaders to areas where they need to concentrate their efforts to change the cultures.

Leaders have also been able to analyze responses about individual questions: "Important issues are well communicated at shift change" is one of these questions. The percentage of respondents who "agree" with this particular statement range from 13 percent to 100 percent. As the survey data continue to be parsed out, by physicians and by nurses, Ascension will have enough information to evaluate the microcultures that occur within individual units.

When asked how Ascension will actually use these data to change the organizational culture, Pryor replied, "Overall I've been told we're 15 to 30 points higher in the distribution than any other organization [Bryan Sexton and colleagues] have surveyed. Even so, it becomes clear at the unit level that there is substantial opportunity for improvement. We've also integrated the work into our national scorecard goals for this year [with goals for each subsequent year] as well. Our goal for this year is that 40 percent of units will score 65 percent or higher on both safety climate and teamwork climate."

Ascension has developed a baseline that will allow the organization to evaluate the data and set goals for the next year or two. The organization is not just saying it wants to be better; it has also established what we refer to at IHI as "how-good-by-when goals."

CONCLUSION

As we think about the cultures we create in our healthcare organizations, we must also think about the mediums for growth that are in place and sustenance of these cultures. Will the mediums for growth that you currently have in place foster the types of cultures needed to achieve your organizational objectives? Taking more time to truly understand your organizational cultures is one of the best things you can do this year.

WHERE TO LEARN MORE

Information on the Safety Climate Survey developed by Bryan Sexton and colleagues can be found at www.ihi.org/IHI/Topics/PatientSafety /MedicationSystems/Tools/Safety%20 Climate%20Survey%20(IHI%20Tool).

REFERENCES

Deming, W. E. 2000. *Out of the Crisis, 1st edition*. Cambridge, MA: The MIT Press.

———. 1993. *The New Economics for Industry, Government, Education*. Cambridge, MA: MIT CASE.

Freiberg, K., and J. Freiberg. 1996. *NUTS! Southwest Airlines' Crazy Recipe for Business and Personal Success*. Austin, TX: Bard Press.

Herzberg, F. 2003. "One More Time: How Do You Motivate Employees?" *Harvard Business Review* 81 (1): 87–96.

Pryor, D. 2005. Personal communication, October 25.

Reinertsen, J. 2005. Personal communication, November 11.

Taber's Cyclopedic Medical Dictionary, 14th edition. 1983. Philadelphia, PA: F. A. Davis Company.

Transform the Discharge Process

"**D**ischarge" should be a dirty word in healthcare. Patients too often experience failures in the process when being transferred from one care setting to another or from the care setting to home. Worse still is the potential harm caused by breakdowns in the discharge process. One of the six interventions recommended by the IHI's 100,000 Lives Campaign is to prevent adverse drug events through mandatory medication reconciliation at every transition in care. This life-saving step is just one aspect of the discharge or transition process that can be improved. In fact, the entire process begs for critical examination and redesign.

An international study on healthcare quality conducted by The Commonwealth Fund (2004) revealed some disturbing trends. Failures to coordinate care during discharge were a common theme that emerged in all six countries studied, with at least one-third of patients saying they received no instructions on the following: ▶

- What symptoms to watch
- Who to contact with questions
- How to get follow-up care

The study also found that medication regimens were especially problematic at the transition points, with 25 percent of patients saying no one reviewed their prehospitalization medications during discharge where they received a new medication regime. The researchers concluded that these gaps in care and continuity cause errors, readmissions, duplicate tests, and the need for the patient to act as a communication bridge between transition points.

BREAKDOWNS AT TRANSITION POINTS

Breakdowns in information transfer are at the heart of the problem. Eric Coleman, M.D., M.P.H., associate professor of medicine in the divisions of Health Care Policy and Research and Geriatrics at the University of Colorado at Denver Health Sciences Center, has conducted research into the care-transition process. In 2004, he found the following problems at transition points:

- Discharge and/or transfer information is inadequate or not conveyed to the next setting.

- Documentation of patient information for transfer purposes (from one hospital to another) is not legible 28 percent of time.
- Advance care directives are unavailable for 75 percent of patients at the time of acute illness.

The consequences of these breakdowns range from simple patient confusion and frustration to dangerous complications in care such as conflicting orders and adverse drug events.

In 2006, Coleman assembled transition-points experiences from both the patient's and clinician's perspectives. This study revealed that patients feel inadequately prepared for the next care setting because they receive conflicting advice about the management of their illness; they are unable to reach the right practitioner to answer their health-related questions; and they are uncertain about their role in self-care after discharge. The study also indicated that it is rare for one clinician to orchestrate patient care across multiple settings and that many physicians have never practiced in settings to which they transfer patients.

Coleman's research reveals a common thread: A properly executed transition or discharge process is a critical element of high-quality care. Far too frequently, however, this process is broken.

EXAMINING READMISSIONS

One way to evaluate the quality of the discharge process is to look at the occurrences of readmissions. If we define a readmission as a failure of discharge preparations, outpatient services, or support for self-management in the community, then we can identify these failures and examine the nature of the breakdown. Roger Resar, M.D., a physician in the Mayo Health System and a member of IHI's Innovation Team, conducted an informal chart review of readmitted patients and found the following reasons for readmission:

- Forty percent were related to the discharge process (50 percent of which were deemed preventable)
- Twenty-seven percent were related to inadequate outpatient services and lack of support at home (85 percent of which were deemed preventable)
- Twenty-three percent were related to separate, distinct disease processes (6 percent of which were deemed preventable)

After examining the 40 percent of readmissions related to the discharge process, Resar (2005) identified the following defects within the discharge process:

- Anticoagulation issues
- No discharge plan
- No long-term care plan
- No description of patient's functional status
- No return appointment scheduled

If readmission is the starting point of failures in care, Resar's review indicates that the main focus of care improvement should be changing the discharge and transition process.

REDESIGNING THE DISCHARGE PROCESS

A hospital team can undertake redesign by first asking key questions; the answers will drive the new design:

- What has to be redesigned (or what needs to be changed)?
  1. Handoffs between staff and family
  2. A new process for discharging patients with special/unique needs

- How may the redesign process begin?

1. Review charts of patients who have been readmitted, and interview patients to identify failures in discharge preparations.
2. Initiate prototype tests to eliminate discharge failures on a nursing unit or a service that is highly likely to successfully implement the changes.
3. Offer support, guidance, ideas, and energy to the prototype unit or area to encourage achievement of significant changes. Then, assign a senior leader the responsibility of spreading the new performance level throughout the organization.

A successful redesign will accomplish the following:

■ Reduce readmissions
■ Meet patient needs and preferences
■ Boost patient and family confidence and comfort level during and after the transfer
■ Meet the needs of clinicians and other practitioners within the community

These suggestions are by no means a comprehensive road map to a successful redesign of the discharge process, but they are an ideal starting point.

Example: TCAB's "Transition Home"

Transforming Care at the Bedside (TCAB) is an innovation project funded by The Robert Wood Johnson Foundation and led by IHI. One of its goals is to improve the quality of care at all transition points. As part of this work, the TCAB team identified a typical patient-care process flow for the "Transition Home," a high-leverage change process aimed at preventing readmissions, adverse events, and mortality that result from failures in the discharge process. The premise of this process is that comprehensive and reliable discharge planning and post-discharge support may reduce readmission rates and improve health outcomes.

The TCAB team came up with the following list of elements that should be included in an ideal design of a patient-care process flow (see Figure 3.1):

■ Early assessment of needs and resources, involving family input
■ Efficient and coordinated discharge process, including scheduling discharge
■ Improved patient understanding of the process using health-literacy principles, such as using written materials, simulation, Teach Back (see Idea 5), and a discharge quiz

Figure 3.1. Idealized Process Flow for the "Transition Home"

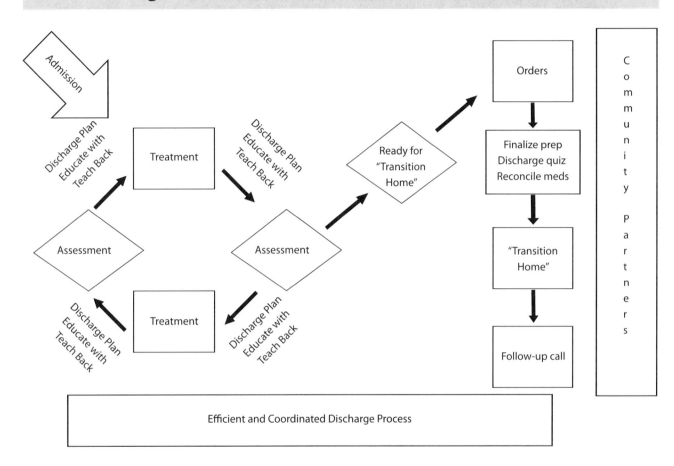

Source: The Robert Wood Johnson Foundation and IHI TCAB Project. Reprinted with permission from Institute for Healthcare Improvement, Cambridge, Massachusetts.

- Comprehensive patient preparation and follow-up, including phone calls to the patient within 24 hours and reconciliation of various patient medications

- Collaboration or partnerships with nursing homes, home health, and community facilities
- Follow-up call and/or appointments with primary care physicians or specialists

Each change made to this idealized process flow involves careful and comprehensive communication between the caregivers and the patient. If incomplete information transfer is one of the key design flaws, then improved communication (at every step) will go a long way toward eliminating that flaw.

In addition, the TCAB team also adopted a tool (originally developed by Virginia Mason Medical Center in Seattle, Washington) called "Ticket Home" that can improve the discharge and transition process. The "Ticket Home" tool is a white board placed at each patient bedside that lists discharge- or transition-related information, including anticipated date and time of discharge, pain management plans, home preparation, social supports, and even details of transportation and subsequent medical visits. Information on the "Ticket Home" board and the discharge plan is entered at admission and is continually updated throughout the care process by the care team, the patient, and the family. As such, the tool becomes part of the daily rounds and the goal-setting process.

The "Ticket Home" board provides transparency about the patient care plan and serves as a constant visual cue about the patient's progress toward achieving key milestones that are required for discharge from the hospital. When everyone—the care team as well as the patient and family—knows the care plan and the status of the patient's progress, the process is likely to go more smoothly and the patient and family will be better prepared for the transition back home.

CONCLUSION

Many of the defects in patient care, including medication confusion, misunderstanding about care protocols, and inadequate preparation at the recovery site, occur at the delicate points of care transfer, when the patient is more vulnerable. These transition points are critical, so properly designed processes should be in place. When clinicians redesign care across handoff points and take on the responsibility of guiding patients across these "white spaces," readmission rates decrease, patients report less anxiety, and overall outcomes are improved.

WHERE TO LEARN MORE

- Coleman, E. A. 2004. "Lost in Transition: Challenges and Opportunities for Improving the Quality of Transitional Care." *Annals of Internal Medicine* 141 (7): 533–36.
- Learn more about the Transforming Care at the Bedside initiative at www.ihi.org/IHI/Programs/TransformingCareAtTheBedside/.
- For more information about the "Ticket Home" board, visit www.ihi.org/IHI/Topics/Medical SurgicalCare/MedicalSurgicalCare General/ImprovementStories/Shes GotaTicketToGoHome.htm.

REFERENCES

Coleman, E. A. 2004. "Transitional Care: Focus on Clinical Care and Quality." Presentation at the National Health Policy Forum meeting. [Online information; retrieved 6/16/06.] nhpf.ags.com/handouts/Coleman.slides_10-07-04.pdf.

———. 2006. "Commissioned Paper: Transitional Care Performance Measurement." Appendix I in *Performance Measurement: Accelerating Improvement*, 250-79, by the Committee on Redesigning Health Insurance Performance Measures, Payment, and Performance Improvement Programs. Washington, DC: National Academies Press.

The Commonwealth Fund. 2004. *First Report and Recommendations of The Commonwealth Fund's International Working Group on Quality Indicators.* New York: The Commonwealth Fund.

Resar, R. 2005. Personal communication, October 27.

Engage in **Dialogue** to Improve Teamwork, Communication, and Patient Safety

In the movie *Cool Hand Luke*, Luke (played by Paul Newman) finds himself in a no-win situation. As the result of a series of unfortunate events, he ends up in a small, southern prison where he and the stern and controlling warden are on an inevitable collision course. Their conflict escalates when Luke emerges as a leader of the inmates, much to the chagrin of the warden and his henchmen. Luke is always bucking the system and, after being put in solitary confinement numerous times and going through a variety of escapades with the guards and ▶

the inmates, the warden finally calls Luke aside and tells him that things are not going as the warden expects. The warden then turns to Luke and utters the classic line, "What we have here is a failure to communicate." But Luke, in his usual cool-hand fashion, does not see things in the same light. Throughout the movie, he tries to create a foundation for an open dialogue with the warden and the guards, something he successfully accomplishes with the inmates.

Figure 4.1 depicts two ways of communication and may explain why there was a "failure to communicate" between Luke and the warden. The warden and his men followed the communication style on the left side of the diagram, or the "old way." This style is characterized by minimal learning, fear, and closed-minded thinking. It creates a defensive posture that discourages new ideas. On the right side of the diagram is the "new way," the style that Luke modeled. This style is characterized by reflection and openness to new ideas, trust, and collaboration, all of which Luke represents when he deals with fellow inmates. Clearly, Luke understands the multiple ways of communication, while the warden has no concept of this notion.

TWO PATHS OF COMMUNICATION

Every time we engage in human discourse, we have options not only for the manner in which we approach the communication (old way versus new way) but also for how to actually structure the details of the exchange. One of the most influential writers on this subject is David Bohm, whose work on dialogue has become an international standard on how to enhance human communication. Bohm (1996) points out in his classic work, *On Dialogue*, that an invitation to have a dialogue comes before two or more individuals get together to exchange information (see Figure 4.2, a composite representing the works of Edgar Schein, William Isaacs, and David Bohm). This invitation, which may be explicit or implicit, leads the participants to a conversation or the opportunity to "turn together." This conversation (or turning together) then moves on to deliberation and that deliberation allows participants to select between two different paths—suspension and discussion.

"Suspension" is characterized by listening and building trust, while "discussion" is characterized by advocating and competing. Unfortunately, most people end up

Figure 4.1. Optimizing Communication: Old Way Versus New Way

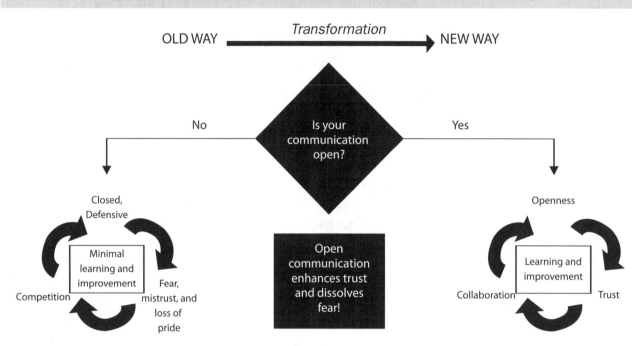

Source: Adapted and reprinted with permission from R. C. Lloyd and Associates.

going down the discussion route, which is where we find the warden and his gang. Along this path are lesser forms of communication: discussion, dialect, and debate— exchanges that position the participants as combatants rather than partners. According to Bohm, the objective of these forms of communication is to put forth your point of view to dominate the views of the others involved in the exchange.

Effective communication is a product of the suspension path, depicted on the left side of Figure 4.2. Accepting the invitation to an exchange entails the suspension of assumptions about the matter at hand and a willingness to explore the theories and predictions about that subject matter. For example, if you are part of an exchange about the value of establishing a rapid response team, do you enter the

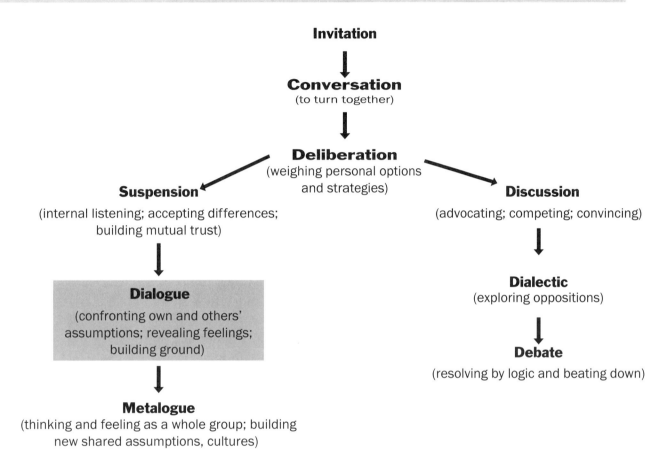

Figure 4.2. A Framework for Dialogue

Invitation

↓

Conversation
(to turn together)

↓

Deliberation
(weighing personal options
and strategies)

Suspension
(internal listening; accepting differences;
building mutual trust)

↓

Dialogue
(confronting own and others'
assumptions; revealing feelings;
building ground)

↓

Metalogue
(thinking and feeling as a whole group; building
new shared assumptions, cultures)

Discussion
(advocating; competing; convincing)

↓

Dialectic
(exploring oppositions)

↓

Debate
(resolving by logic and beating down)

Source: Adapted and reprinted with permission from R. C. Lloyd and Associates.

exchange with preconceived ideas about the merits of such a team, or do you approach the subject with an open mind and willingness to consider alternative perspectives?

Once you go through the initial process of suspension, you can easily move into the actual dialogue, where both parties address assumptions and set the stage for the final step in the communication cascade: the metalogue. "Metalogue," a term coined by Bohm, is the process of agreement, where both parties think and feel as a group, build new shared assumptions, and form a new culture.

Bohm (1985, 175) summarizes the stages of dialogue as follows:

> [It is] an awakening.... [T]he process of dialogue itself is a free flow of meaning among all the participants. In the beginning, people were expressing fixed positions, which they were tending to defend, but later it became clear that to maintain the feeling of friendship in the group was much more important than to hold any position. Such friendship has an impersonal quality in the sense that its establishment does not depend on a close personal relationship between participants. A new kind of mind thus begins to come into being which is based on the development of a *common meaning* that is constantly transforming in the process of the dialogue.

According to Bohm (1996), the following are characteristics of a dialogue:

- Opposition is minimized.
- Participation in the "pool of common meaning" is increased.
- Constant development and change guide the words of the participants.

- No preestablished purpose is brought to the meeting, and new purposes may emerge.
- No member is excluded, and no particular content is excluded.
- Consciousness of the nature of relationships arises.
- Transformation of relationships occurs.
- A dialogue begins but does not end.

These characteristics are very different from those that typify discussions, conversations, and meetings that occur regularly in healthcare organizations.

Dialogue elevates not only your own understanding of meaning but also the other party's understanding. In almost all of his writings, Bohm points out that although there is a beginning to a dialogue, there is really no end to learning how to dialogue.

EXAMPLE: OSF ST. JOSEPH MEDICAL CENTER

Bohm's ideas on communication have been making their way into the healthcare environment, as this example illustrates.

OSF St. Joseph Medical Center in Bloomington, Illinois, turned to dialogue after it studied the results of the root cause analyses it conducted. The analyses identified a poor system of communication as a proximal cause of more than 90 percent of the system's adverse events. According to Kathy Haig (2005), director of quality resource management, patient safety officer, and risk manager at OSF St. Joseph:

Misinterpretation of verbal and written communication among healthcare providers is a major concern and a common occurrence in healthcare today. JCAHO notes that 65 percent of sentinel events include communication as a contributing factor. At OSF St. Joseph Medical Center we found that communication is a factor in 90 percent of the root cause analyses [we] conducted. A lack of structure and standardization for communication, in addition to variations in communication style, can lead to differing "mental models" between caregivers or not "hearing" what is actually being said.

The team at OSF St. Joseph learned that people were talking to each other, but they were not really understanding what was being said. In short, the medical center was a primary candidate for a dialogue. The medical center used a dialogue technique called SBAR, which stands for Situation-Background-Assessment-Recommendation. The origins of SBAR can be traced back to the aviation industry, where it is used in Crew Resource Management, which is a series of briefings, debriefings, and trainings to ensure the identification of conditions that may negatively affect the flight crew's ability to fly a successful mission. The SBAR tool is used (in aviation or in healthcare situations) to communicate a potentially complex and dangerous event in a brief and standardized format.

In healthcare, the use of SBAR has allowed professionals to more effectively evaluate the status of a patient and to provide recommendations that are clear and unambiguous. An example of how the SBAR technique is used is shown in Figure 4.3, which illustrates communication between a doctor and a nurse about a critical patient situation. Haig explains the multilayered benefits brought on by the medical center's use of SBAR:

A surgeon was upset about receiving extraneous phone calls from the nursing unit. A new process was

Figure 4.3. Example of Using the SBAR Technique to Establish a Dialogue

S*ituation* (Whats going on?)	"I'm calling about Mr. Smith. He is short of breath."
B*ackground* (What are the important facts?)	"He's a patient with chronic lung disease. He's been sliding downhill, and he's now actually worse."
A*ssessment* (What do you think is the problem?)	"He has decreased breath sounds on the right side. I think his lung has probably collapsed."
R*ecommendation* (What do you suggest or request?)	"I think he probably needs a chest tube. I need you to see him now."

Source: Reprinted with permission from Institute for Healthcare Improvement, Cambridge, Massachusetts.

immediately developed in which the staff put their concerns in SBAR format. The upshot of the process change is that the surgeon stated, "I don't know what you did, but it worked." Staff members are encouraged to make "recommendations" based on their observations, and this not only assists the physician with situational awareness through the eyes of the bedside caregiver but also empowers frontline staff by having input [into] and influence over decisions in the management of the patient's care. The use of SBAR in both oral and written communication has improved patient safety by providing concise, clear, [and] accurate information in an organized format between caregivers. In short, SBAR is a wonderful tool to help nurses talk more like doctors and help doctors listen more like nurses.

EXAMPLE: PARK NICOLLET HEALTH SERVICES

Another example of how dialogue improves healthcare practice is illustrated in this story about Park Nicollet Health Services in Minneapolis, Minnesota. David Wessner, president and chief executive officer of Park Nicollet, and his leadership team invited employees to a dialogue around two issues on the strategic plan: (1)

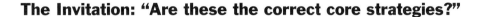

Figure 4.4. Creating a Foundation for Dialogue at Park Nicollet Health Services

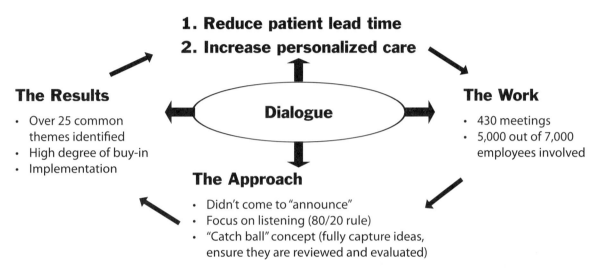

The Invitation: "Are these the correct core strategies?"

1. Reduce patient lead time
2. Increase personalized care

Dialogue

The Results
- Over 25 common themes identified
- High degree of buy-in
- Implementation

The Work
- 430 meetings
- 5,000 out of 7,000 employees involved

The Approach
- Didn't come to "announce"
- Focus on listening (80/20 rule)
- "Catch ball" concept (fully capture ideas, ensure they are reviewed and evaluated)

Source: Used with permission from Park Nicollet Health Services, Minneapolis, Minnesota.

reducing patient lead time (i.e., waits for appointments and in physicians' offices) and (2) increasing personalized patient care.

Figure 4.4 shows the dialogue process created by the management team at Park Nicollet to enable more than 5,000 associates and physicians to explore their assumptions, ideas, and thoughts about the strategic objectives. To ensure that every stakeholder in the organization had input and a voice in the dialogues, more than 430 meetings were scheduled. Members of the management team facilitated the

sessions, using the "80/20 rule"—that is, talk 20 percent of the time and listen 80 percent of the time, because listening sets the context for dialogue.

More than 25 common themes emerged from these sessions, enabling the management team to go back to the strategic objectives and to figure out what had to be achieved, when it had to be achieved, and how to achieve it. Ultimately, the organization created an entirely new framework for developing a culture that values the art of dialogue.

Wessner articulates his enthusiasm for what the dialogue has accomplished in his organization:

> We set out to ask every staff member whether ideas for breakthrough, hatched in the planning process, would work for their patients and for them. The resulting dialogue exceeds our expectations, and we are way ahead in tapping every person's energy for what we need to do next year.

CONCLUSION

To improve our understanding of communication, among ourselves and with our patients, we need to learn alternatives to the usual approaches to human discourse. The works of Bohm, Isaacs (1993), and Schein (1993) provide the conceptual foundation for such knowledge. Developing dialogue skills with practical tools such as the SBAR technique and strengthening the ability to manage "difficult conversations" (Stone, Patton, and Henn 1999) should help healthcare professionals avoid being confronted with that classic line, "What we have here is a failure to communicate."

WHERE TO LEARN MORE

- For more information about the SBAR technique, visit www.ihi.org/IHI/Topics/PatientSafety/SafetyGeneral/Tools/SBARTechniqueforCommunicationASituationalBriefingModel.htm.
- Senge, P. M. 1990. *The Fifth Discipline*. New York: Currency Doubleday.

REFERENCES

Bohm, D. 1985. *Unfolding Meaning: A Weekend of Dialogue with David Bohm*. Loveland, CO: Foundation House.

———. 1996. *On Dialogue*. New York: Routledge.

Haig, K. 2005. Personal communication, October 31.

Isaacs, W. N. 1993. "Taking Flight: Dialogue, Collective Thinking, and Organizational Learning." *Organizational Dynamics* (Autumn): 24–39.

Schein, E. H. 1993. "On Dialogue, Culture, and Organizational Learning." *Organizational Dynamics* (Winter): 40–51.

Stone, D., B. Patton, and S. Henn. 1999. *Difficult Conversations*. New York: Penguin Books.

Teach the New Language of
Health Literacy

Most of us can recall situations in which jargon, complex directions, unfamiliar words, and the resulting stress of semantics got in the way of a service we were either receiving or giving. Many times, such misunderstandings cause breakdowns in healthcare—a patient who fails to take a medication "as ordered" or who did not "respond to treatment" is an example. As the Institute of Medicine (2004) report, *Health Literacy: A Prescription to End Confusion*, states, "health literacy is fundamental to quality care." It is necessary to teach a new language of "health literacy" to ensure that patients and families do not suffer needlessly from avoidable communication breakdowns and have a better understanding of health information and medical-care instructions.

PATIENTS AT RISK

Health literacy is a predictor of health status (Baker et al. 2002). In fact, research shows that literacy is a stronger predictor of health status than age, income, ▶

employment status, education level, or racial and ethnic group (Schillinger et al. 2002). Some of the negative outcomes that can stem from limited health literacy include the following (Williams et al. 1998; Baker 1999; Baker et al. 2002; Scott et al. 2002):

- Lower likelihood of receiving preventive services
- Limited knowledge of chronic conditions
- Poor asthma self-care
- Higher utilization of services
- Worse health outcomes

The scope of health illiteracy is staggering. Someone who is functionally literate enough to cope with most other aspects of life can still struggle mightily with understanding medical instructions and orders. According to estimates, as much as half of the U.S. population are health illiterate and, as such, are at risk of misunderstanding medication instructions and improperly following care directions, both of which result in excess hospitalizations and generally poor health outcomes. While mistakes and misunderstandings are frustrating and embarrassing in other aspects of life, in healthcare they can be dangerous and even deadly.

Why are so many people, even those who have adequate or functional literacy, at risk? There are several reasons. First, healthcare relies heavily on the written word. Medications are dispensed along with a print-out of related information, including dosage, instructions, side effects, and dangers of interactions with other drugs. For patients who struggle with reading, receiving this information only in written form heightens their risk. This overreliance on the written word extends beyond medication dispensation. A caregiver might decide to put a patient on a strict diet. If the instructions are conveyed only in writing, the patient who cannot read well will have enormous difficulty following the diet.

Second, healthcare options have rapidly grown, including the number of medications available today. As doctors prescribe an increasing variety of new medications, patients can find themselves confused about which drugs treat which conditions. While someone with functional literacy may be able to find out about a new drug on the Internet, patients who struggle with reading have fewer options for additional information. Often, these patients turn to untrained family members and friends for help in deciphering complex medical or medication orders. Caregivers must provide simple and clear verbal instructions to such patients.

Similarly, new tests and procedures have arisen for old health problems. This trend is problematic for the health illiterate because it relies on patient involvement. Although involvement of patients in their own care generally leads to improved outcomes, it requires more responsibility from patients. Patients who have limited or inadequate health literacy are increasingly at risk because they do not have complete understanding of their role in the self-care process. As more healthcare organizations adopt the principle of patient involvement as a core tool for improvement, caregivers must recognize and fill the crucial need for clearly communicating care expectations to patients and asking patients to demonstrate their understanding of those expectations.

Third, healthcare is rife with jargon. Perhaps, it is rightfully so; after all, medicine is a complicated subject with its own language. Jargon causes few negative consequences when it is used between two parties (e.g., two pharmacists) who are both conversant in it. But when it is understood only by one party in a two-way exchange (e.g., a pharmacist and a patient), jargon can be dangerous. For example, a team at Iowa Health System in Des Moines studied health literacy in their healthcare system. The team found that more than 80 percent of communication between staff and patients involved the use of jargon; less than 20 percent was jargon-free. Imagine a patient who has been treated for hypertension for years but has never been told that hypertension means high blood pressure. Such a scenario might seem almost ridiculous, but it does happen, even though it is easily preventable. The use of jargon only adds a level of unnecessary complexity to an already complex conversation. It is well within the capacity of all healthcare staff to simplify the language and terminology they use to communicate with patients, and they should be encouraged to do so.

TEACH BACK

Caregivers should always consider whether or not the patient they are talking to has the capacity to understand all aspects of the conversation. Effective communication and demonstrated understanding between patient and caregiver are both crucial elements of high-quality care. "Teach Back" is one technique that can help the caregiver communicate effectively and be assured that the patient understands. It is an elegantly simple concept: After the caregiver communicates instructions to the patient, the caregiver then asks the patient to explain or "teach back" what he has just been informed to do.

The Teach Back method not only increases the caregiver's confidence that the patient properly understands the instructions, it also serves as a feedback mechanism for the caregiver, letting the caregiver know if the instructions lack clarity so that she can take steps to improve the explanation. As clinical staff go through repeated iterations of communicating instructions to patients and asking for teach back, they will note which communication strategies and methods work best. They will also become more knowledgeable about how instructions are interpreted by different groups of patients and then be able to tailor those instructions to improve the reliability of patient understanding.

Some of the critical elements of care that patients should be asked to teach back are as follows:

- The importance of keeping the follow-up visit
- Self-care on return home
- Contact information for getting help, if needed
- Use and doses of prescribed medications

Research is revealing the benefits of Teach Back. According to the Agency for Healthcare Research and Quality (2001) report *Making Health Care Safer*, "Asking that patients recall and restate what they have been told" is one of 11 top patient safety practices based on strength of scientific evidence. In addition, a study specifically related to diabetic patients shows that physicians' application of interactive communication to assess patient recall or comprehension—a process known as "closing the loop"—was associated with better glycemic control for diabetic patients (Schillinger et al. 2003).

The need for using non-shaming language with patients is important when employing the Teach Back technique. Patients who struggle with literacy too often interpret this technique as a "test" for the healthcare system to blame or shame them for not understanding medical instructions. In fact, caregivers are the ones who are responsible for helping each patient understand and should tailor instructions based on individual needs. The *Joint Commission 2006 Requirements Related to the Provision of Culturally and Linguistically Appropriate Health Care* specifically address this caregiver responsibility; the guidelines include the following:

- The caregiver must respect the patient's right to and need for effective communication.
- The caregiver must give the patient
  - education and training specific to needs and appropriate to care, treatment, and services; and
  - education and training specific to abilities.
- The caregiver must transfer or discharge the patient based on assessed needs and the hospital's capabilities.

Example: Iowa Health System

The Joint Commission guidelines help caregivers at the Iowa Health System in Des Moines understand the importance of asking each patient on admission, "How do you learn best—written materials, videos, or talking face-to-face?"

As a test of the Teach Back method, staff called congestive heart failure (CHF) patients at two different times—both at 48 hours and at one week after discharge—to ask how they weighed themselves and to clarify patient understanding of the correct method. Staff noticed a disturbing level of variation. Some patients weighed themselves fully dressed one day and then undressed on another day. Other patients weighed themselves before breakfast one day and then after breakfast the next. In addition, staff found that 48 hours after discharge, only about half of the CHF patients were weighing themselves in accordance with instructions. This variation caused confusion for both patients and staff. When a team at Iowa Health examined reasons for readmissions of CHF patients, the team found that this variation was a primary contributing factor to readmission.

A week after the first staff check-in with CHF patients and after patients participated in Teach Back, staff found that about 78 percent of patients were weighing themselves correctly. These results not only show the effectiveness of the Teach Back method, they also demonstrate the need to use this technique continually throughout the care process. Repeated requests for patients to demonstrate understanding evidently increase their chances of fully comprehending and complying with medical instructions. Therefore, using Teach Back as a regular communication tool, not only at discharge, is critical in providing high-quality care.

ASK ME 3

Like Teach Back, Ask Me 3 is an attractively simple tool to improve communication with patients so they fully understand care instructions. This technique uses three simple questions that cover three crucial elements of understanding a medical condition and its care: (1) diagnosis, (2) treatment, and (3) context. The three questions are:

1. What is my main problem? (Diagnosis)
2. What do I need to do? (Treatment)
3. Why is it important for me to do this? (Context)

This tool benefits both the patient and the caregiver. Ask Me 3 works under the assumption that the caregiver anticipates these three questions, whether or not the patient actually asks them. Indeed, if the patient has to ask, then the communication from the caregiver is clearly inadequate. This technique involves the caregivers putting themselves in the position of the patient and tailoring the communication to ensure that the three key questions are discussed clearly and satisfactorily. Teaching the Ask Me 3 technique to patients and families also presents the added benefit of increasing the reliability that healthcare professionals use all three components to support patient understanding of care instructions.

SIMPLIFIED FORMS

The final idea for addressing limited health literacy is to ensure that the forms patients must complete are clear in their instructions and intent. An example of this idea in practice comes from Iowa Health, where a team identified a problem of unclear consent forms. Following is a portion of the old consent form:

> I authorize _____Hospital to retain, preserve and use for scientific, teaching or commercial purposes, or to dispose of at their discretion, any specimens or tissues removed from my body. I release to _____

Hospital all of my ownership interests or other rights to these specimens, tissues or other materials.

In collaboration with adult learners, Iowa Health rewrote the form to simplify the language, remove the jargon, and increase overall clarity. The revised consent form text follows:

I understand the doctor may remove tissue or body parts during this surgery or procedure. If it is not used for lab studies or teaching, it will be disposed of, as the law requires.

This idea is an important example of how all aspects of staff-to-patient communication, both verbal and written, need to be simplified to properly and clearly inform (and hence care for) the patient.

CONCLUSION

Literacy, whether functional or health related, is a delicate subject. Feelings of shame and embarrassment will inevitably emerge when addressing this issue with patients who may have limited ability to read and write. However, this should not discourage caregivers from addressing a patient's potential problem with literacy. In fact, caregivers must take into account this factor to provide appropriate care and clearly communicate information. Effective communication with all patients is a key element of good care; failure to establish effective communication contributes to poor outcomes.

Nearly all patients struggle with "health literacy," regardless of their ability to read and write. The complexity of healthcare and healthcare professionals' reliance on using medical jargon and terminology create problems for all patients in understanding and following care instructions. The ideas and tools discussed here can serve as starting points for addressing the problems of health literacy and improving communication between caregivers and patients.

WHERE TO LEARN MORE

- For more information on improving patient understanding and promoting clear communication, visit the Pfizer Clear Health Communication website at www.pfizerhealthliteracy.com/.
- For the U.S. Department of Health and Human Services' "Quick Guide to Health Literacy," visit www.health.gov/communication/litera cy/quickguide/healthinfo.htm.

REFERENCES

Agency for Healthcare Research and Quality. 2001. *Making Health Care Safer: A Critical Analysis of Patient Safety Practices*. Evidence Report/Technology Assessment, Number 43. AHRQ Publication No. 01-E058. [Online information; retrieved 6/28/06.] www.ahrq.gov/clinic/ptsafety/pdf/ptsafety.pdf.

Baker, D. W. 1999. "Reading Between the Lines: Deciphering the Connections Between Literacy and Health." *Journal of General Internal Medicine* 14 (5): 315–17.

Baker, D. W., J. A. Gazmararian, M. V. Williams, T. Scott, R. M. Parker, D. Green, J. Ren, and J. Peel. 2002. "Functional Health Literacy and the Risk of Hospital Admission Among Medicare Managed Care Enrollees." *American Journal of Public Health* 92 (8): 1278–83.

Institute of Medicine. 2004. *Health Literacy: A Prescription to End Confusion*. Washington, DC: National Academies Press.

Joint Commission on Accreditation of Healthcare Organizations. 2006. *Joint Commission 2006 Requirements Related to the Provision of Culturally and Linguistically Appropriate Health Care*. [Online information; retrieved 6/28/06.] www.jointcommission.org/NR/rdonlyres/1401C2EF-62F0-4715-B28A-7CE7F0F20E2D/0/hlc_jc_stds.pdf.

Schillinger, D., K. Grumbach, J. Piette, F. Wang, D. Osmond, C. Daher, J. Palacios, G. D. Sullivan, and A. B. Bindman. 2002. "Association of Health Literacy with Diabetes Outcomes." *JAMA* 288 (4): 475–82.

Schillinger, D., J. Piette, K. Grumbach, F. Wang, C. Wilson, C. Daher, K. Leong-Grotz, C. Castro, and A. B. Bindman. 2003. "Closing the Loop: Physician Communication with Diabetic Patients Who Have Low Health Literacy." *Archives of Internal Medicine* 163 (1): 83–90.

Scott, T. L., J. A. Gazmararian, M. V. Williams, and D. W. Baker. 2002. "Health Literacy and Preventive Health Care Use Among Medicare Enrollees in a Managed Care Organization." *Medical Care* 40 (5): 395–404.

Williams, M. V., D. W. Baker, E. G. Honig, T. M. Lee, and A. Nowlan. 1998. "Inadequate Literacy Is a Barrier to Asthma Knowledge and Self-Care." *Chest* 114 (4): 1008–115.

Implement
WalkRounds™
to Identify and
Address Safety Issues

The Patient Safety Leadership WalkRounds™ concept was developed by Dr. Allan Frankel, director of patient safety at Partners HealthCare in Boston (Frankel et al. 2005). It is a leadership tool designed to enhance the culture of safety within an organization, incorporating frontline insights into operational decisions and as such guaranteeing feedback loops to the staff and to the board. It provides (1) a structured method for leaders to talk with frontline staff about safety issues in the organization and (2) a rigorous mechanism to analyze information, identify effective actions, and ensure they are performed.

The WalkRounds process is very different in intent, methods, and outcomes from clinical rounds or customer service rounding that most healthcare professionals conduct. A core group (including senior executives, board members, and/or ▶

vice presidents) conducts weekly visits to different departments of the hospital. The group talks with one or two nurses and other available staff from the department to ask specific questions about adverse events or near misses within that area and about the factors or systems issues that led to these events. The group then analyzes the information and takes action to address the issues identified.

Organizations that have sponsored WalkRounds have discovered two major benefits of this practice:

1. Frontline staff appreciate that their concerns are heard and are acted on by management.
2. Board leaders gain insight into quality and safety concerns that they were not previously aware of and see that actions are taken to proactively reduce the probability of adverse events.

TWO COMPONENTS: CONVERSATION AND DATA

WalkRounds have two major components. The first is the conversation component, a carefully choreographed dialogue between frontline staff and the following people:

- A hospital leader (or two)
- A patient safety officer/manager/director/specialist
- A scribe
- Others (e.g., managers, pharmacists, residents, as deemed appropriate)

This dialogue lasts about one hour and can be repeated regularly, based on the urgency of the identified issues or the amount of follow-up required. Typically, WalkRounds are scheduled as frequently as weekly, but at a minimum monthly. The conversations can be held wherever frontline staff do their work (e.g., care units, pharmacy, labs). They should not be held in a senior leader's office or in a room reserved for management meetings. The objective is to get leaders and staff to meet where the real work on the unit or in the department is done.

If the conversation component provides the rich content of WalkRounds, then the data component provides the foundation for action. Figure 6.1 illustrates the specific aspects of the data component. During the conversation stage, the scribe serves as the data collector. After the dialogue, the scribe turns the quantitative and qualitative findings into reports that will be

Figure 6.1. The Data Component of WalkRounds™

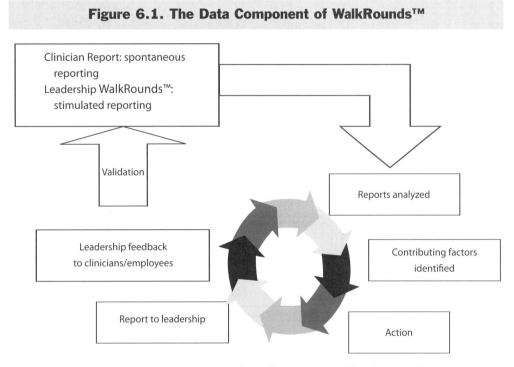

Source: Adapted and used with permission from Allan Frankel, M.D., Boston, Massachusetts.

reviewed by the team that conducted the WalkRounds. The team then documents the factors that have been contributing to the safety concerns identified by staff and develops action strategies.

The team presents a summary report at the regular leadership meeting, and the leaders who conducted the WalkRounds follow up with the department's frontline staff and appropriate clinicians. The reports and action plans validate the process and provide the impetus to conduct more WalkRounds.

EXAMPLE: SAFER PATIENTS INITIATIVE

WalkRounds have been an integral part of the Safer Patients Initiative (SPI) in the United Kingdom for more than two years and provide a good example of how cultural transformation can be advanced through dialogue. The SPI work is funded through the London-based Health Foundation, and the program activities are directed and facilitated by IHI. The overall goal of this effort is to reduce adverse events in four primary National Health Service (NHS) trusts by 50 percent over four years. The four trusts include Conwy and Denbighshire in Wales; Luton and Dunstable Hospital in England; NHS Tayside in Scotland; and Down Lisburn Health and Social Services in Northern Ireland. The use of WalkRounds has increased steadily within these trusts, and the practice is now the cornerstone for the cultural and leadership components of SPI.

The 80/20 Rule

David Gozzard, M.D., chief medical officer, and Annette Bartley, director of quality and patient safety, provide executive leadership for the SPI WalkRounds at Conwy and Denbighshire NHS Trust. Their visits to the wards typically involve about 10 to 12 people. They visit with a list of thought-provoking questions in hand to stimulate the dialogue; more likely than not, however, staff are ready with their own lists of issues to discuss. A hallmark of the Conwy and Denbighshire WalkRounds is that it follows the 80/20 rule, which David Wessner and his team also

used in their dialogue sessions with staff at Park Nicollet Health Services (see Idea 4 for details).

Gozzard and Bartley talk 20 percent of the time and listen 80 percent of the time. They talk about issues related to patient safety and quality, including the culture of safety, medication administration, and housekeeping services. Other issues not related to patient safety and quality (e.g., availability of parking, employee benefits, or vacation schedules) that creep into the conversation are not ignored but are placed on a list of items to be addressed in another meeting. Remember that the focus of WalkRounds is strictly on patient safety and quality, and nothing else.

Good Housekeeping

A wonderful example of how staff get involved with WalkRounds is provided by Iona Davies, a member of the housekeeping staff at Conwy and Denbighshire. During one of the sessions, Davies brought a large pile of papers to the WalkRounds gathering and explained how she and the housekeeping staff had redesigned the room-cleaning process. They brainstormed a list of 21 items that needed to be cleaned in a consistent and standard manner after a patient was discharged. Their objective was to establish a reliable room-cleaning process that is safe, is efficient, is effective, and contributes positively to the flow of patients in the discharge process.

To standardize the new process, leaders developed a check sheet that included the 21 items submitted by the housekeeping staff (i.e., clean bed frame, cables and wires, and furniture and equipment; restock gloves and alcohol gel; empty and clean patient locker; and so on). Every housekeeper was given training in the use of this check sheet: the staff member who cleaned the room has to sign the sheet and leave it on the bed for the next patient to see. This sheet is a way to let the next patient know that each housekeeper has a personal commitment to guaranteeing that the room is properly cleaned and prepared.

Although it may seem like a small thing to some, the check sheet is a clear demonstration by the leadership team at Conwy and Denbighshire that the safety and quality concerns of the housekeeping staff are as important to them as the issues brought up by physicians and nurses. The WalkRounds sessions also pointed out other issues that could not have been identified independently by the management team; these concerns came from the people who deliver care at the front lines every day:

- Staffing. Where this has been a significant threat to patient safety, management has intervened and ensured appropriate coverage
- Environmental issues. For example, plugs needed and trailing cables, hazardous steps, seating that is too low for elderly patients
- Oversedation. This was highlighted in gastro patients, and the team is now formulating local guidelines that will reduce variation in sedation administration dosage and be based on national guidance
- Quality of preparation of inpatients for emergency endoscopic procedures
- Audiology. Test-room doors weighed half a ton and opened out onto the corridor

CONCLUSION

WalkRounds assist management and staff in their efforts to transform the organization's culture, particularly toward a focus on patient safety and quality. Organizations that have been successful at implementing WalkRounds acknowledge two key learning points:

1. When used with "Safety Briefings" (another improvement tool), WalkRounds help leaders achieve success in creating and emphasizing a safety culture better than either tool used alone.
2. Leaders who focus solely on safety concerns during WalkRounds are more successful at creating a culture of safety than leaders who use the visits to discuss a variety of topics, such as budgets and patient satisfaction.

WHERE TO LEARN MORE

- Learn more about developing a culture of safety, including how to implement WalkRounds and Safety Briefings, by visiting www.ihi.org/ IHI/Topics/PatientSafety/Medicati onSystems/Changes/Develop+a+ Culture+of+Safety.htm.
- Tools for conducting WalkRounds are available at www.ihi.org/ IHI/Topics/PatientSafety/SafetyGe neral/Tools/Patient + Safety + Lead ership + WalkRounds(tm) + %28IH I + Tool%29.htm.
- Tools for conducting Safety Briefings are available at www.ihi .org/IHI/Topics/PatientSafety/ MedicationSystems/Tools/Safety% 20Briefings%20(IHI%20Tool).
- For more information on the Safer Patients Initiative, visit www.ihi .org/IHI/Programs/SaferPatientsIni tiative/.
- Budrevics, G., and C. O'Neill. 2005. "Changing a Culture with Patient Safety Walkarounds." *Healthcare Quarterly* (Special Issue 8): 20–25.
- Frankel, A. (ed). 2006. *Strategies for Building a Hospitalwide Culture of Safety*. Chicago: Joint Commission Resources. Available at http://store.trihost.com/jcaho/ product.asp?dept%5Fid = 34&cata- log%5Fitem = 741.

REFERENCE

Frankel, A., S. P. Grillo, E. G. Baker, C. N. Huber, S. Abookire, M. Grenham, P. Console, M. O'Quinn, G. Thibault, and T. K. Gandhi. 2005. "Patient Safety Leadership WalkRounds™ at Partners HealthCare: Learning from Implementation." *Joint Commission Journal on Quality and Patient Safety* 31 (8): 423–37.

Move from Patient Satisfaction to the Ideal Patient Experience

R esearch shows that involving patients in clinical decision making and care design produces better outcomes and enhances patient satisfaction at a lower cost. Despite this reality, patients still routinely report that staff seem too busy and are too focused on the routines of providing care rather than on the patients' unique and specific needs during their hospital visit or stay.

The Institute of Medicine (IOM 2001) established six "aims for improvement" in its report *Crossing the Quality Chasm*, paying attention to the need for patient-centeredness. Putting the patient at the center of care goes beyond mere patient satisfaction. Patient-centeredness does not mean just listening to the patient's voice (too often captured only in a survey) but rather making the patient's voice the centerpiece of any effort to evaluate or redesign care. ▶

Four of IOM's "simple rules" support this move to patient-centeredness:

1. Customization based on patients' needs and values
2. The patient as a source of control
3. Shared knowledge and free flow of information
4. Evidence-based decision making

THE PATIENT'S VOICE AS THE DRIVER FOR CHANGE

Patient-satisfaction surveys may satisfy rules 1 and 3, but they fail to take advantage of the patient as a source of control. Determining whether a patient was satisfied with the quality of care he received is a far cry from using the patient's voice as the driver for change and improvement. Furthermore, rarely do patient-survey results lead to redesigns that will meet the IOM aims. A patient-centered design uses both the evidence from science and the needs and desires of the patient in creating a complete model of care.

The idea is to move from ensuring patient satisfaction to creating the ideal patient experience. The challenge of designing care for each patient may be daunting for many physicians and nurses. However, segmentation and innovative tools are available that can take away the assembly-line approach to care and usher in a designed care experience in a way that also makes the lives of healthcare professionals more rewarding. Four innovative ideas developed independently in various care settings will help in customizing care:

1. Diabetes visit cards
2. Lauren's List
3. Daily goals and multidisciplinary rounds with patients
4. Decision aids

DIABETES VISIT CARDS

Successfully treating diabetes, or any chronic disease, depends on the patient's adoption of a specific, often strict, set of guidelines for everyday behavior. Caregivers often feel handcuffed because they simply cannot control (or even successfully monitor) the behavior of the patient outside the care setting. They can establish guidelines and carefully explain the reasons for their recommendations and orders, but, ultimately, the responsibility for maintaining health lies with the patient.

Better clinical outcomes are achieved when diabetic patients are more involved in planning their care. With this premise in mind, the Design Council in the United Kingdom developed diabetes visit cards for the Bolton Hospitals NHS Trust. Figure 7.1 shows a sample set of these cards.

Each card presents a common issue faced by patients with diabetes —for example, managing exercise routines, making healthy lifestyle choices, monitoring vital measures, and making appropriate clinical decisions. At the start of a doctor's visit, the patient is given an entire deck of cards from which the patient can select six to eight cards that most accurately convey the problems she is facing regarding diabetes treatment. The nurses and physician use these selected cards to determine the agenda for the patient visit.

This simple idea conveys not only that the patient's voice is being heard but also that the caregivers are attuned to the specific, unique needs of the patient at that particular visit. The patient, as a result, feels more involved and has a better sense of ownership of her treatment. As the patient gains experience and confidence in her own care and confronts new

challenges about her illness, caregivers can include a discussion about the cards as a regular part of the visit, ensuring an open and effective dialogue for each interaction.

As a result of the implementation of these cards, outcomes have improved and patient satisfaction is extremely high at this hospital.

LAUREN'S LIST

This innovative idea was developed by Lauren, a young patient who suffered from a chronic gastrointestinal disease that made her a frequent visitor to the hospital. Frustrated with her care and the loss of control she experienced with each hospitalization, Lauren taped to the door of her hospital room a piece of paper that listed three requests for any caregiver who came to see her. In time, Lauren refined her list. Ultimately, the hospital adopted Lauren's idea for use by all patients, creating a placard that is placed around the door handle to patients' rooms that lists four simple instructions:

1. Please knock and wait for my reply.
2. Please introduce yourself.

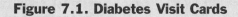

Figure 7.1. Diabetes Visit Cards

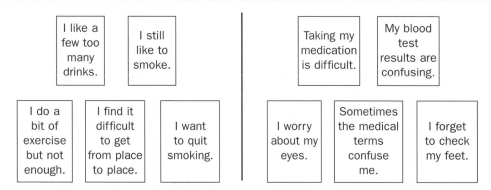

| I like a few too many drinks. | I still like to smoke. | | Taking my medication is difficult. | My blood test results are confusing. |
| I do a bit of exercise but not enough. | I find it difficult to get from place to place. | I want to quit smoking. | I worry about my eyes. | Sometimes the medical terms confuse me. | I forget to check my feet. |

Source: Adapted from Design Council, London, England, and Bolton Hospitals NHS Trust, Bolton, England.

3. Please discuss with me why you are here.
4. Please tell me if something might hurt.

The development and implementation of Lauren's List holds many lessons for healthcare leaders and caregivers who are looking to create the ideal patient experience. No lesson is clearer, however, than the imperative of listening to the patient, restoring patient control, and decreasing patient anxiety whenever possible. Research shows that efforts to minimize patient stress, noise in the hospital, and patient anxiety have a positive impact on outcomes of care (Ulrich et al. 2004).

DAILY GOALS AND MULTIDISCIPLINARY ROUNDS WITH PATIENTS

The nursing staff at Seton Northwest Hospital in Austin, Texas, conduct regular nursing rounds not only as a means to detect patient distress early (see Idea 1) but also as a way to create the ideal patient experience. Like many other ideas presented by Reinertsen and Schellekens (2004) and Bisognano and Plsek (2006), this idea can yield better outcomes without the need to add staff or capital expense to the unit budgets.

Regular rounds that involve physicians, nurses, and patients are becoming standard practice. Two key elements to these multidisciplinary rounds create a superior patient experience. First, patient goals are established by the entire team each day in the context of monitoring progress toward discharge and beyond. Second, these goals and active progress measurements are clearly documented on a white board affixed at each patient's bedside. Documenting goals and progress and displaying these prominently for each patient has facilitated positive, productive communication among staff, patients, and family members. The patients, participating in the design of the day, are making the goals a priority.

DECISION AIDS

This idea comes from work being conducted by Albert G. Mulley, M.D., M.P.P., at Massachusetts General Hospital in Boston. Treatment options for certain clinical conditions are not clearly supported by medical evidence. The best decisions in these cases often are based on shared decision making and consider patient preferences and values. For example, the treatments for benign prostatic hyperplasia and breast cancer—conditions for which medical evidence is unclear and the implications of care options have a profound impact on the patient's life—represent areas for shared decisions.

Decision aids are tools used in the shared decision-making process that allow patients to make more informed decisions about their care options. These aids are often video-based and conducted in conjunction with nurse coaching to help patients make the best decisions on care. Because patient values often play a role in these decisions, decision aids should include tools that allow for discussion of values that affect treatment choices. The proper use of decision aids requires both training and support. However, the improved outcomes and generally lower costs achieved by the use of decision aids (O'Connor, Llewellyn-Thomas, and Flood 2004) justify the required training time and costs.

CONCLUSION

Creating an ideal patient experience can be done in an infinite number of ways, and the ideas presented here offer just some of the possibilities. We hope these ideas will get you thinking about new ways to improve the patient experience in your own care setting. As you work on improving the care experience for patients, be sure to keep the patient at the center of both your mind and your designs.

REFERENCES

Bisognano, M., and P. Plsek. 2006. *10 More Powerful Ideas for Improving Patient Care*. Chicago: Health Administration Press and the Institute for Healthcare Improvement.

Institute of Medicine, Committee on Quality of Health Care in America. 2001. *Crossing the Quality Chasm: A New Health System for the 21st Century*. Washington, DC: National Academies Press.

O'Connor, A. M., H. A. Llewellyn-Thomas, and A. B. Flood. 2004. "Modifying Unwarranted Variations in Health Care: Shared Decision Making Using Patient Decision Aids." *Health Affairs* (Suppl Web Exclusive): VAR63–72.

Reinertsen, J. L., and W. Schellekens. 2004. *10 Powerful Ideas for Improving Patient Care*. Chicago: Health Administration Press and the Institute for Healthcare Improvement.

Ulrich, R., C. Zimring, X. Quan, A. Joseph, and R. Choudhary. 2004. "The Role of the Physical Environment in the Hospital of the 21st Century: A Once-in-a-Lifetime Opportunity." [Online information; retrieved 9/14/06.] www.healthdesign.org/research/reports/pdfs/role_physical_env.pdf.

Redesign Care
to Be More Responsive
to Patient Needs

There are basically two approaches to making a process more responsive to customer needs and expectations:

1. The process improvement approach is based on the assumption that the current process is fundamentally sound and can be retained. The objective for improvement, therefore, is to make incremental and constant improvements to the existing process by reducing variation and increasing the reliability of the process.

2. The process redesign approach, on the other hand, starts with the assumption that the current process is fundamentally broken and not capable of meeting (let alone exceeding) customer wants, needs, and expectations. In this case, ▶

the objective is to completely redesign the process from the ground up. The output of the process may remain the same, but the steps, work assignments, and physical layout of the redesigned process may bear little resemblance to the original process.

Much of what has been classified as quality improvement in healthcare has been incremental process improvement rather than fundamental process redesign. Redesign requires a different way of thinking, a different set of tools and approaches, and a different level of motivation. Unfortunately, when healthcare professionals do attempt to redesign a process, they are frequently met with resistance and statements such as, "Oh, that will never work," "Do you realize what you are asking?", or "That idea requires entirely too much change."

REDESIGN IS EVERYWHERE

Photocopying is a primary example of redesign. It was not too long ago when photocopiers did not exist; if you wanted to make a copy of a document, you used carbon paper while typing or you cut a stencil and placed the master on a mimeograph machine and turned a manual crank to churn out copies. If you were lucky, you had a motorized mimeograph machine, which was quite the technological advancement. Today we throw a document into the copier, hit a few buttons, and pull out 100 copies, collated and stapled, in a matter of minutes. We do not even think about it.

Automated Teller Machines (ATMs) provide another classic example of a redesigned process. Today most people do not use bank tellers to process their transactions; they use ATMs or a drive-up convenience station. When banks first started offering ATM services, people did not use them because it was not the way banking was done. Gradually, however, as a result of good marketing and society's intolerance for waiting, the ATM caught on and rapidly became a standard way of banking.

Consider a clinical example of redesign that we now take for granted. There was a time when cataract surgery required a five- to seven-day stay in the hospital. The patient's head was stabilized with sandbags on either side, and the entire procedure was a delicate matter. Today cataract surgery is performed on an outpatient basis, and patients are able to see shortly after the procedure is completed.

The point is that many aspects of life have been redesigned. The question is, what aspects of healthcare need to be further redesigned and how should such efforts be structured and implemented?

IHI's Idealized Design Model (Moen 2002), shown in Figure 8.1, provides a framework for organizing the components of redesign and thinking about what it takes to become fully engaged in either the design of a new process or system or the redesign of an existing process or system. The model has three major components: generate new ideas, test new ideas, and spread new ideas. These major components are then divided into five phases that guide the actual work of a design or redesign team.

GENERATE NEW IDEAS

This component is Phase 0 of the Idealized Design Model. At this point, the team is generating new ideas about how the process or system could be designed or redesigned. The team screens, observes, and then synthesizes ideas from many quarters to determine which new ideas will be most appropriate. Site visits to other types of industries might also be part of this initial phase. Once the team completes these steps, it should conduct a milestone meeting to make sure that the new ideas align with the overall aim and purpose of the team's work.

TEST NEW IDEAS

Phase 1 of the model is the planning phase, in which the team begins to define the nature and scope of the new product, process, or service. In Phase 2, the team actually specifies the design for the new product, process, or service. This may require different skill sets and knowledge than those used in Phase 1, depending on the nature of the redesign effort. Content experts should be invited to team meetings to fill the knowledge gaps as they can serve as periodic consultants to the redesign team or be part of the team on an ongoing basis.

Phase 3 is the prototype testing stage. It involves conducting initial tests of the new design on a small scale. These are tests for learning that should allow the team to gain a better understanding of the ability of the new design to meet the design

Figure 8.1. IHI's Idealized Design Model

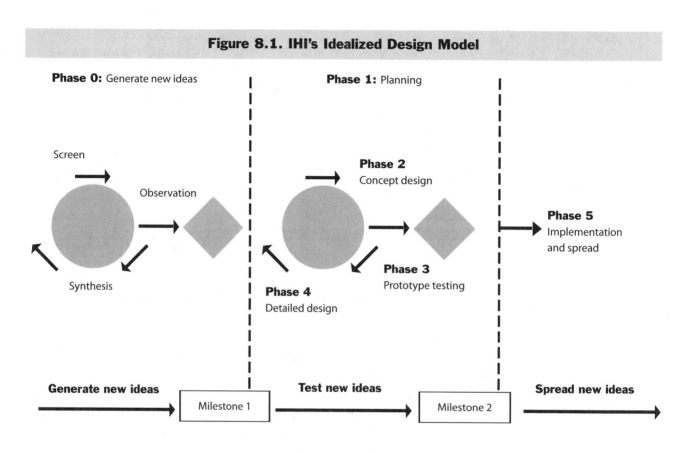

Source: Reprinted with permission from Institute for Healthcare Improvement, Cambridge, Massachusetts.

targets and the overall aim. Revisions from this initial testing are then taken to the next phase.

Phase 4 is when the team engages in detailed testing; the robustness of the design should become apparent at this stage. This is the time for testing the design components under different conditions to determine if the new ideas, procedures, products, or services are able to consistently produce the same results. At the conclusion of Phase 4, the team should conduct another milestone meeting to evaluate how the work progressed through Phases 1 through 4 and what revisions need to be made to either the design or the components of the design before moving on to spread the ideas.

SPREAD NEW IDEAS

Phase 5 is the stage that many people want to move to as soon as they have identified the need for change. However, many teams do not achieve the desired outcomes because they failed (1) to note the differences between implementation and spread, and (2) to properly structure the activities needed to guarantee successful implementation and spread.

The key distinctions between these key terms are as follows:

- *Implementing* a change is making a change a part of the day-to-day operations of an area, unit, or department.
- *Spreading* a change is disseminating the change beyond the initial team's work area.

EXAMPLE: CLINICA CAMPESINA

One organization that has success-fully used the Idealized Design Model is Clinica Campesina. With three locations in north central Colorado, Clinica Campesina Family Health Services serves more than 25,000 patients. Sixty percent of its patients are Hispanic, 70 percent are uninsured, and 100 percent are medically underserved. Led by CEO

Pete Leibig, medical affairs vice president Carolyn Shepherd, and IHI project director Cory Sevin, Clinica Campesina has completely redesigned its care delivery processes and demonstrated dramatic improvements over time.

The organization started its redesign journey (the idea-generating phase) by thinking about how it could improve its services. Initially, it thought it could engage in simple, incremental improvement, but it quickly realized the need to abandon the existing ways of delivering care and to fundamentally redesign the process. For example, the team analyzed the existing office layout and concluded that it was not customer friendly, restricting the flow of work. The team then took the standard office configuration and converted it into a completely new layout based on pods.

The team realized that the old process was a "shuffle process," in which patients checked in at the main reception desk, sat in the waiting area, and moved or shuffled (depending on the number of patients that day) from room to room until finally able to see their doctors. The redesign entailed creating three pods, a dentistry pod, and a waiting area, as shown in Figure 8.2.

Figure 8.2. Clinica Campesina Layout

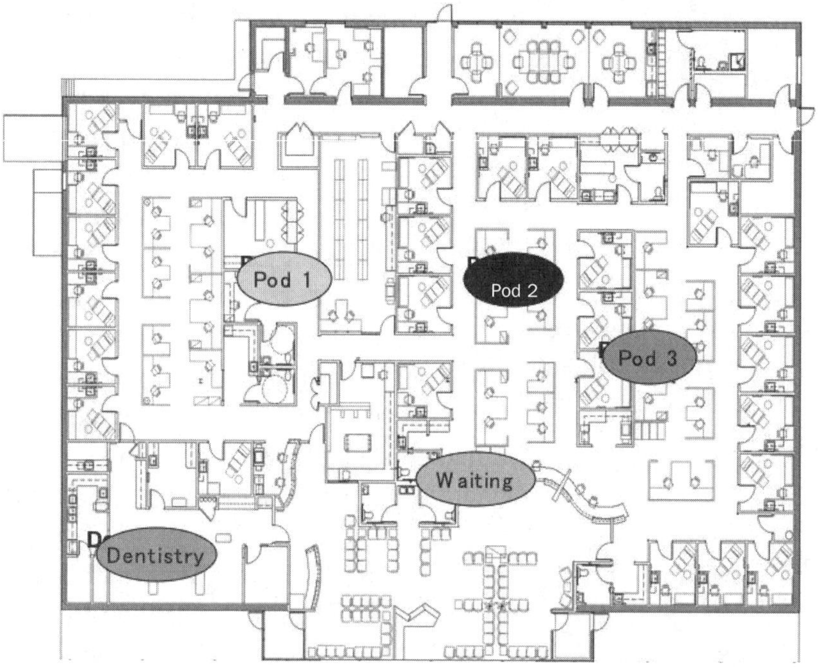

Source: Reprinted with permission from Clinica Campesina, Lafayette, Colorado.

Each pod is serviced by upwards of 13 professionals, who come to the patient instead of having the patient come to them. The patient comes to the appropriate pod and essentially experiences one-stop shopping. Within the pod, the patient is registered, receives care, schedules follow-up visits, receives financial information, and arranges for transportation home if needed.

As a result of this fundamental redesign (which included changes in work assignments, work processes, work roles, and physical plant modifications), Clinica Campesina has seen dramatic improvements in process and outcome measures. The following areas benefited greatly from the redesign effort:

- *Appointment no-shows* (see Figure 8.3): In 1999, the baseline rate of appointment no-shows was 36 percent. In January 2005, after the redesign, the no-show rate declined to 8 percent, and the rate has remained at or slightly below this percentage since then.

Figure 8.3. Clinica Campesina Redesign Results: No-Show Appointments

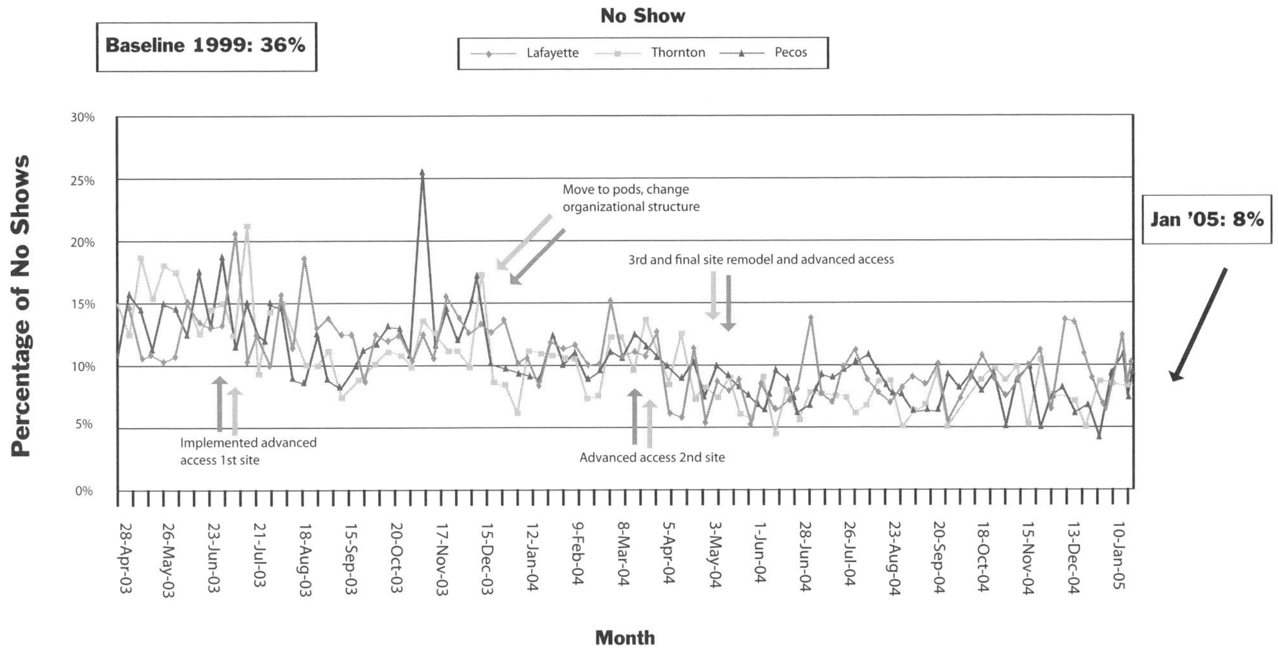

No Show

Baseline 1999: 36%

| ◆ Lafayette | ▪ Thornton | ▲ Pecos |

Jan '05: 8%

Move to pods, change organizational structure

3rd and final site remodel and advanced access

Implemented advanced access 1st site

Advanced access 2nd site

Percentage of No Shows

Month

Source: Reprinted with permission from Clinica Campesina, Lafayette, Colorado.

■ *Access to care:* Before the redesign, the clinic was providing care to about 14 patients per full-time equivalent (FTE) per day. After the redesign, it was able to accommodate more patients, providing care to more than 18 patients per FTE per day. This improvement occurred while the state of Colorado was instituting a series of budget cuts for health service providers. While Clinica Campesina was losing revenue from the state, it was able to make up for the losses by increasing volume and being more efficient by instituting open access and improving the flow of care in the office.

■ *Disease management:* Clinica Campesina was able to observe a gradual increase in the continuity of care, across all sites that offered asthma care; the increase ranged from 64 percent to 87 percent.

■ *Immunizations* (see Figure 8.4): Improving the percentage of children 2 years of age and younger who receive appropriate immunizations has been a key

Figure 8.4. Clinica Campesina Redesign Results: Immunizations

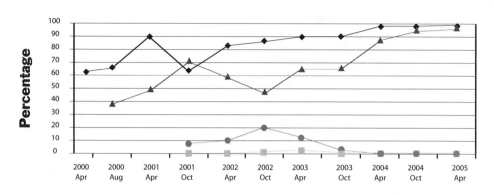

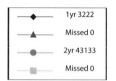

Source: Reprinted with permission from Clinica Campesina, Lafayette, Colorado.

measure of organizational success for several years. As a result of the redesign, Clinica Campesina has seen a constant increase in the percentage of children receiving their shots and a comparable reduction in the percentage of missed shots.

LESSONS LEARNED

Clinica Campesina's experiences with redesign are not atypical. Realizing that incremental improvement will not move the organization to its desired breakthrough levels is a motivating factor in a redesign effort. What must be clear to organizations seeking to redesign a product, process, or service, however, is the fact that old habits die hard. When organizations engage in redesign, it quickly becomes clear to them that

the people aspect of the effort is a more difficult set of variables to manage than the rearrangement of physical structures and space.

Key lessons in redesign efforts include the following:

- Systems thinking is the foundation for redesign. If the interactions of all the parts of a process or system are not considered, the redesign effort will be nominal at best.
- A team approach is essential. Redesign requires highly functional teams that have the will, ideas, and ability to properly execute the design concepts.
- Clear and detailed documentation of the team's decisions, measures, progress reports, and resource allocations is critical. Documentation

allows accurate and timely updates on progress, evaluation of performance over time, and capture of all required resources to inform future redesign efforts.

- Measurement plays a central role throughout the redesign process. It is also critical afterwards to ensure that the gains are held.
- Teams need knowledge and skills in a variety of quality improvement tools and techniques.
- The organization must allocate sufficient time, effort, and resources to the redesign effort. Successful redesign cannot occur if team members are expected to dedicate 100 percent of their time and energy to the redesign work in addition to their full-time job responsibilities.
- Redesign usually takes longer to complete than other incremental improvement efforts.

CONCLUSION

Perhaps the most challenging aspect of redesign is changing the mind-set about the work and establishing new ways of doing the work. Redesign is the ultimate test of an organization's true will to change; this is why many teams avoid engaging in redesign. Some organizations may claim to be redesigning some aspects of the work, but on closer look, they are at best doing incremental improvements. That redesign seems entirely too complicated and risky and requires too much work to make it succeed leads teams to do what is easy instead of what is right.

Redesign requires more time, more effort, and a new mind-set. It includes changing the culture and engaging in a new dialogue.

WHERE TO LEARN MORE

- For more information about setting aims for improvement, establishing measures, and selecting and testing changes, visit www.ihi.org/IHI/Topics/ Improvement/ImprovementMetho ds/HowToImprove/.
- To learn more about spreading changes, see:
  - "Spreading Changes" at www.ihi.org/IHI/Topics/Improv ement/SpreadingChanges/.
  - "A Framework for Spread" at www.ihi.org/IHI/Results/White Papers/AFrameworkforSpread WhitePaper.htm.

REFERENCE

Moen, R. 2002. *A Guide to Idealized Design.* [Online information; retrieved 6/16/06.] www.ihi. org/IHI/Topics/Improvement/ImprovementMethods/Literature/AGuidetoIdealizedDesign.htm.

Accelerate Improvement with Orchestrated Tests of Change

P DSA, or Plan-Do-Study-Act, cycles are familiar to most of those engaged in healthcare improvement work. The value of using this methodology—conducting rapid tests of change on a small scale by planning a change, testing it, observing the results, and acting on what is learned—has been well established, and the practice has been widely adopted. Yet improvement in healthcare is not progressing quickly enough. Often, staff who are initially excited about improvement work get discouraged by the seemingly endless rounds of redesigning and evaluating without achieving the intended results. Given the critical importance of improving healthcare quickly, new ideas and new tools to speed up this process can help.

One promising approach to testing new ideas is called "orchestrated testing." This idea stems from the project Transforming Care at the Bedside (TCAB), ▶

a collaboration between IHI and The Robert Wood Johnson Foundation. Ron Moen, lead faculty member on the project and an expert in process improvement, and Pat Rutherford, the project director, worked with TCAB teams to identify problems associated with the standard, one-test-at-a-time improvement methodology and set out to improve it. The sites in the TCAB project tested the orchestrated testing approach.

BENEFITS OF ORCHESTRATED TESTING

Orchestrated testing allows for improved test design—better replication, randomization, and standardization. In addition, because orchestrated testing allows for more than one change to be tested at the same time, it enables a multiple-factor design approach that also examines the interaction between changes. Most importantly, orchestrated testing results in more learning, with fewer resources required, and at a faster pace. All these improvements do not come without a cost, however; testing multiple changes at once is inherently more complex and requires a leader with improvement expertise and experience to oversee the orchestration

of improvement efforts. The increased attention to improvement efforts through simultaneous tests of changes is repaid by faster and deeper results.

LEARNING FROM THE ORCHESTRA

How this new methodology is "orchestrated" is important to understand. Figure 9.1 shows the elements of an orchestra and its corollaries in an orchestrated test design. Perhaps the most important thing to note about this illustration is the role of the improvement advisor, or IA.

An IA provides day-to-day leadership, helping to identify, plan, and execute improvement projects throughout the organization; deliver successful results; and spread changes throughout the entire system. IAs must have advanced knowledge and skills in the art and science of improvement, as well as the ability to work with and coach frontline teams in achieving and maintaining successful changes. IAs are always crucial to process redesign and testing, but in the orchestrated testing methodology they are particularly important as the

Figure 9.1. Elements of an Orchestra Correlated to Elements of an Orchestrated Test

Orchestra	Orchestrated Test
Multiple sections: wind, brass, string	Multiple test sites that are all different
Led by a conductor who sets and maintains the tempo (speed); dynamics; and interpretation, including articulating style	Improvement advisor acts as the conductor
All sections cooperate in the service of music making (sometimes some players are resting, not playing)	Each site signs up to test specific changes
All members of the orchestra agree to standardize and tune to a specified pitch	All sites agree to the specified changes and the test plan
The orchestra rehearses and performs	Improvement advisor calls all sites before, during, and after the tests of change; all sites carry out the tests as planned
All sections contribute to the whole; no performance is given if any section is missing	All sites must complete their tests to have a successful orchestrated test, and each site gets more out of the orchestrated test than they put into its specific test

Source: The Robert Wood Johnson Foundation and IHI TCAB Project. Reprinted with permission from Institute for Healthcare Improvement, Cambridge, Massachusetts.

conductor of multiple, simultaneous changes.

Figure 9.2 shows the differences between the single-change testing method and the orchestrated multiple-change testing method.

EXAMPLE: ORCHESTRATED TESTING IN TCAB

TCAB proved to be a natural testing ground for orchestrated tests, because it involved multiple sites

Figure 9.2. A Comparison of Single-Change and Multiple-Change Testing Methods

	Testing a Single Change	Testing Multiple Changes Simultaneously
One site	Single-factor experiment (common)	Multiple-factor experiment (rare)
Multiple sites (current)	Each site selects its own change on its own test schedule	Subject-matter expert "bundles" a set of changes to be tested as a single factor
Multiple sites (proposed)	Each site selects the same change and tests it on the same schedule ("fast-track test")	Each site does one multiple-change test on the same schedule ("orchestrated test")

Source: The Robert Wood Johnson Foundation and IHI TCAB Project. Reprinted with permission from Institute for Healthcare Improvement, Cambridge, Massachusetts.

that joined together for a multiyear project to achieve dramatic improvements in care at the bedside and in the working environments on medical-surgical units. Rather than each site developing its own plans and informing the other sites, the entire group collaboratively designed the portfolio of tests needed for rapid change. With the guidance of the IA, the teams set out to test this portfolio of changes simultaneously.

Four changes were proposed for the orchestrated test by the TCAB sites. Figure 9.3 describes the four changes and lists who was required for the test and what the test involved.

Once the design for each individual test has been established, the next step in the orchestrated test approach is to look at the tests as individual "instruments" in a larger "orchestra." The TCAB orchestrated test was designed such that each site tested two assigned changes for one month. The sites in this case are the 13 pilot sites that participated in Phase 2 of the TCAB project. (Two of the TCAB sites did not conduct tests.)

Only one site tested all four changes during the month; this was, in itself, another test. By having sites test different combinations of changes, with one site testing all four changes at once, the TCAB design team was able to evaluate the advantages and disadvantages of conducting tests

Figure 9.3. Orchestrated Test of Multiple Changes in TCAB Sites

Change	Who	What
Test 1: Assess competency levels of frontline staff using SBAR (Situation-Background-Assessment-Recommendation) through scenario-based training	Registered nurses on the unit	• The nurses will be trained in SBAR • After the SBAR training, competency will be assessed using case-based scenarios
Test 2: Use checklists to capture key patient data at handoffs (change of shift or multidisciplinary daily rounds)	Nurses and other providers participating in handoffs or rounds	A standardized checklist will be used at either change of shift or multidisciplinary daily rounds (depending on involvement in Test 4)
Test 3: Train all frontline staff in how to have "difficult conversations"	All nurses (including registered nurses and licensed practical nurses)	• Staff will be trained, using *Difficult Conversations* material (Stone, Patton, and Henn 1999) • Staff will complete the two-page worksheet on a difficult conversation they experienced recently • If possible, staff will practice with someone with whom they are having a difficult conversation
Test 4: Institute true multidisciplinary daily rounds (include nurses, physicians, and other key staff at the bedside)	Nurses, doctors, and key ancillary providers	• Daily rounds at the patient bedside will incorporate a discussion of the patient goals for the day, projected discharge date, and clinical planning • Patients and families will be involved in the discussion

Source: The Robert Wood Johnson Foundation and IHI TCAB Project. Reprinted with permission from Institute for Healthcare Improvement, Cambridge, Massachusetts.

of different numbers of changes simultaneously.

Before conducting this orchestrated test in the TCAB project, the IA established the following parameters, which are useful to any facility that is considering this test design:

- All four changes must be standardized so that they are the same for all sites.
- Each site must test their assigned set of changes with the same staff group, not test each change separately on different staff groups.
- Each site must complete its assigned test during the same month.
- The four changes must not be in place prior to the orchestrated test.
- No other changes are to be tested during the month.

CONCLUSION

The concept of orchestrated testing is still in its early stages; it is essentially its own test of a strategy for testing changes. However, signs that improvements in testing design can produce deeper and faster results are promising. Organizations may achieve similar results by devoting more resources, both in terms of numbers of people and the amount of time they commit to improvement projects (although both resources are in short supply in healthcare today). Despite the fact that orchestrated testing is a more complex way of laying out hypotheses and managing simultaneous tests of changes, it can produce deep results; this is why this method is so attractive to those trained and involved in improvement work. This new strategy holds promise for teams at sites, such as those involved in the TCAB project, that are seeking to hasten the testing of new ideas. It may also accelerate the process to identify the changes that lead to more rapid improvement.

WHERE TO LEARN MORE

- Learn more about the Transforming Care at the Bedside project at www.ihi.org/IHI/Programs/Transf ormingCareAtTheBedside/.
- For more information on designing tests and the PDSA rapid cycle testing methodology, visitwww.ihi .org/IHI/Topics/Improvement/Imp rovementMethods/HowToImprove/.

REFERENCE

Stone, D., B. Patton, and S. Henn. 1999. *Difficult Conversations: How to Discuss What Matters Most*. New York: Penguin Books.

Establish Red Rules to Increase Reliability

The healthcare industry is known for its large volume of rules—formal written rules as well as informal verbal rules that managers and supervisors establish on a regular basis. In fact, healthcare is flooded with so many rules that staff frequently question them: "Is this a hard and fast rule, or is it a general guideline?" "How much leeway do we have with this rule?" "What will happen if I don't follow this rule?" "Can we modify the rules?" and "Can we create new rules?"

"Red rules" are the three to four key behaviors or practices that staff must follow reliably and accurately to reduce the probability of harm to the patient. These rules should be clearly defined and designed to prevent misunderstanding or ambiguity on the staff's part. E. C. Simpson, a retired executive from the nuclear industry, is generally credited for developing the red-rule procedures. The primary guidelines for establishing red rules are as follows:

- They are few in number.
- They are clear and firm in identifying the consequences for noncompliance. ▶

Cassy Horack (2005), director of patient safety and quality at OSF Saint Francis Medical Center in Peoria, Illinois, explains that "a red rule is something that, except in a rare, urgent situation, we should be doing every time it is indicated within a particular process of caring for a patient." According to Carole Stockmeier (2005), director of the Sentara Safety Initiative at Sentara Healthcare in Norfolk, Virginia, "The power of red rules is the opportunity to focus employee attention on the most safety-critical acts and elevate those acts to ingrained work habits to achieve the highest level of compliance and reliability."

EXAMPLES: OSF SAINT FRANCIS MEDICAL CENTER AND SENTARA HEALTHCARE

Figures 10.1 and 10.2 list the red rules in place at OSF Saint Francis Medical Center and at Sentara Healthcare. Note that, at both organizations, the number of red rules is kept to a minimum. The reason for this is that a long list of red rules (e.g., more than five) can dilute the effectiveness of the rules to the point that they contribute to ambiguity and confusion.

At OSF Saint Francis, the four red rules (Figure 10.1) address clinical aspects of care. At Sentara, red rules (Figure 10.2) are established for both clinical and nonclinical departments. The one red rule that is common between the two organizations is "the operating room timeout," or the Joint Commission requirement that a clinical team takes a timeout at the start of every operation. This rule has received national attention and is implemented in a wide variety of ways in hospitals across the country. Including the timeout as a red rule sends a very clear message: not only is this practice expected, but noncompliance to this practice is unacceptable.

The ventilator red rule at Sentara (i.e., ventilators shall be plugged into red emergency outlets) combines the red rule principle with another important concept in patient safety: intuitive design. In this case, Sentara marked the wall outlets as well as the ventilator plugs with red tape to serve as a visual cue for the staff to match up the color-coded plug with the same-color wall outlet.

Another red rule at Sentara is related to "lock out and tag out," an extension of a strict rule in place in the nuclear and manufacturing

Figure 10.1. Red Rules at OSF Saint Francis Medical Center

Service Area	Red Rule
Central line insertion	Maximal sterile barrier will be established
Circumcision	Analgesia must be used during the procedure
Invasive procedures	Clean surgery scrubs will be available in all areas
Operating room	Timeouts shall be performed prior to all procedures

Source: Reprinted with permission from OSF Saint Francis Medical Center, Peoria, Illinois.

industries. This rule requires that the worker assigned to service or repair a particular piece of equipment shuts the machine down, locks it out so that it cannot function any more, performs the required maintenance, and then unlocks the machine before it can be restarted and used again. As a safety precaution, no other personnel can unlock and start the machine except the individual who initially locked it and tagged it.

Noncompliance Issues

One of the major questions that arise with the introduction of red rules is, "What do we do about noncompliance?" Organizations that have been successful at establishing and implementing red rules have also developed a system for ensuring compliance and have announced their noncompliance policy to physicians, nurses, and support staff.

For example, at Sentara the leadership emphasis is on reinforcing and building strong practice habits around red rules and on reducing the burden to comply. The key component of noncompliance is that the individual knew the rule and made a conscious decision to violate it. If there has been a violation of a red rule:

- The manager is responsible for determining the cause of the violation:
  - Was it an unintended slip or lapse?
  - Did a process problem lead to an unintended slip or lapse?

Figure 10.2. Red Rules at Sentara Healthcare

Service Area	Red Rule
Respiratory services	Ventilators shall be plugged into red emergency outlets
Engineering	Machines and electrical equipment must be locked out and tagged out during service or maintenance activities by the same person
Operating room	Timeouts shall be performed prior to all procedures

Source: Reprinted with permission from Sentara Healthcare, Norfolk, Virginia.

- – Was the employee noncompliant with the red rule?
- The definition for noncompliance is that employees know the rule but still make a conscious decision not to follow that rule.

If an employee is found to have made a choice to act against a red rule, the corrective action is a minimum of a written warning—a consequence that falls midway in the existing performance management program. According to Stockmeier, "Red rules are one tool for aligning beliefs around safety-critical acts and building reliability in performance; it is not a punishment program. There should be no punishment for unintended slips and lapses."

John Whittington (2005) at OSF Saint Francis offers a short and succinct statement about the consequences of noncompliance at his organization: "Noncompliance leads to a visit with the CEO and members of the medical executive team. The medical executive team passed the red rules."

COMPLIANCE SUCCESS FACTORS

Establishing red rules is easy. The factor that determines whether or not the red rules are followed is the fact that leaders of the organization have engaged in a dialogue to assess not only the criteria for determining noncompliance but also the disciplinary actions to be taken when violations occur.

Organizations that have been successful at implementing red rules have identified the following key success factors:

- Thoughtful preparation is required.
- Define only a few rules (three to four).
- Rules must be clear, discrete, and decision-based.
- There must be a clear connection between red rules and safety-critical actions and behavior.
- Focus on recognizing employees for compliance with red rules rather than auditing to catch those who violate the rules.
- Creating red rules is a process of continuous learning and communication.

CONCLUSION

If you are serious about creating a culture of safety in your organization, you need to engage in dialogues (not debates or discussions) about what you intend to achieve and the methods and tools for achieving your aim. Red rules are one of the critical tools for cultural transformation.

WHERE TO LEARN MORE

- Marx, D. 2001. "Patient Safety and the 'Just Culture': A Primer for Health Care Executives." [Online article; retrieved 6/12/06.] www.mers-tm.net/support/Marx_Primer.pdf.
- National Patient Safety Agency, United Kingdom. 2003. "The Incident Decision Tree: Guidelines for Action Following Patient Safety Incidents." [Online information; retrieved 6/12/06.] www.npsa.nhs.uk/site/media/documents/760_IDT%20Information%20and%20Advice%20on%20Use.pdf.
- Reason, J. T. 1997. *Managing the Risks of Organizational Accidents*. Brookfield, VT: Ashgate.

REFERENCES

Horack, C. 2005. Personal communication, September 23.

Stockmeier, C. 2005. Personal communication, October 3.

Whittington, J. 2005. Personal communication, October 6.

ABOUT THE AUTHORS

Maureen Bisognano is the executive vice president and chief operating officer of the Institute for Healthcare Improvement (IHI) in Cambridge, Massachusetts. She is responsible for management of the Institute's many programs and oversees all operations, program development, and strategic planning for IHI. In doing so, she advises healthcare leaders around the world. She is an unrelenting advocate for the needs of patients and is a passionate crusader for change.

Prior to joining IHI, Ms. Bisognano was senior vice president of The Juran Institute, where she consulted with senior management on the implementation of total quality management in healthcare settings. Before that, she served as chief executive officer of the Massachusetts Respiratory Hospital in Braintree, Massachusetts, where, as part of the National Demonstration Project, she introduced total quality management. Her accomplishments in this organization include implementation of the quality improvement program throughout all levels of the hospital.

Ms. Bisognano began her career in healthcare in 1973 as a staff nurse at Quincy City Hospital in Quincy, Massachusetts. She holds a bachelor of science degree from the State University of New York and a master of science degree from Boston University.

Robert Lloyd, Ph.D., is executive director of performance improvement for IHI, providing leadership in the areas of performance improvement strategies, statistical process control methods, development of strategic dashboards, and quality improvement training. He also serves as faculty for various IHI initiatives and demonstration projects in the United States and abroad.

Before joining IHI, Dr. Lloyd served as the corporate director of quality resource services for Advocate Health Care and as director of quality measurement for Lutheran General Health System. In addition, he directed the American Hospital Association's Quality Measurement and Management Project and served in various leadership roles at the Hospital Association of Pennsylvania. Dr. Lloyd received his bachelor's degree in sociology, his master's degree in regional planning, and his doctorate degree in rural sociology from The Pennsylvania State University.

Dr. Lloyd has addressed more than 450 national and international meetings of professional groups and associations. He has served as faculty for organizations, including the American College of Healthcare Executives, the American Society for Quality, JCAHO, and the Group Practice Improvement Network.

He has published articles and reports on a wide range of topics, including CQI theory and implementation, clinical outcomes, and customer satisfaction. Dr. Lloyd is coauthor of the internationally acclaimed book, *Measuring Quality Improvement in Healthcare: A Guide to Statistical Process Control Applications* (ASQP, 2001). He is also the author of *Quality Health Care: A Guide to Developing and Using Indicators* (Jones and Bartlett, 2004).

ACKNOWLEDGMENTS

This book is the result of the work of countless health professionals across the United States and around the world. From Honolulu to Hackensack, from Jönköping to Cape Town, thousands of healthcare leaders, many in executive offices and many on the front lines, deserve our thanks. We are grateful for their commitment to our shared mission to improve the quality of healthcare.

We are indebted to Dan Schummers whose contributions to the writing and management of every detail have made this book possible.

The authors also wish to thank Val Weber and Jane Roessner for their invaluable contributions to the writing and editing of this volume.

A special note of thanks goes to Don Berwick and every member of our amazing staff at the Institute for Healthcare Improvement. In addition, we acknowledge the vital contributions of Tom Nolan, Carol Haraden, Pat Rutherford, Andrea Kabcenell, Kevin Nolan, Ron Moen, Roger Resar, Frank Federico, Terri Simmonds, Fran Griffin, Diane Jacobsen, Marie Schall, Allan Frankel, Kathy Duncan, Lloyd Provost, John Whittington, Joe McCannon, and the entire 100,000 Lives Campaign team—Tami Merryman, Jim Reinertsen, Wim Schellekens, Ann Hendrich, Helen Bevan, Sorrel King, Jane Murkin, Henry Gompertz, David Pryor, Eric Coleman, Kathy Haig, David Wessner, Gail Nielsen, Mary Ann Abrams, David Gozzard, Annette Bartley, Iona Davies, Al Mulley, Lauren, Sally Sampson, Cory Sevin, Pete Leibig, Carolyn Shepherd, Cassy Horack, and Carole Stockmeier.